The Politics of Size

The Politics of Size

Perspectives from the Fat Acceptance Movement

Volume 2

Ragen Chastain, Editor

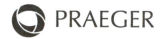 PRAEGER

AN IMPRINT OF ABC-CLIO, LLC
Santa Barbara, California • Denver, Colorado • Oxford, England

Copyright © 2015 by Ragen Chastain

Library of Congress Cataloging-in-Publication Data

The politics of size : perspectives from the fat acceptance movement / Ragen Chastain, editor.
 2 volumes ; cm
 Includes bibliographical references and index.
 ISBN 978–1–4408–2949–9 (hard copy : alk. paper) — ISBN 978–1–4408–2950–5 (ebook)
1. Overweight persons—Health and hygiene. 2. Overweight persons—Social conditions.
3. Overweight persons—Psychology. 4. Fat-acceptance movement. I. Chastain, Ragen, editor.
RC552.O25P64 2015
613.2′5—dc23   2014014311

ISBN: 978–1–4408–2949–9
EISBN: 978–1–4408–2950–5

19 18 17 16 15   1 2 3 4 5

This book is also available on the World Wide Web as an eBook.
Visit www.abc-clio.com for details.

Praeger
An Imprint of ABC-CLIO, LLC

ABC-CLIO, LLC
130 Cremona Drive, P.O. Box 1911
Santa Barbara, California 93116-1911

This book is printed on acid-free paper ∞

Manufactured in the United States of America

The information in this book is not intended to recommend or endorse particular medical treatments or organizations, or substitute for the care or medical advice of a qualified health professional, or used to alter any medical therapy without a medical doctor's advice. For those reasons, we recommend that readers follow the advice of qualified health care professionals directly involved in their care. Readers who suspect they may have specific medical problems should consult a physician about any suggestions made in this book.

Contents

INTRODUCTION

Perspectives on Perspective

Ragen Chastain

When I was approached by Praeger to create this anthology I was thrilled. I knew immediately that I wanted to put together a work that truly explored as many perspectives as possible from the Fat Acceptance movement. I set out to create an anthology that was intersectional in its scope, including People of Color, queer people, people with disabilities, diverse ages, women, men, and Trans* people, and including pieces written by those inside and outside of academia.

Much of the stigmatizing, shaming, and oppression that fat people experience is based on stereotyping. In truth fat people are as diverse as any group of people who share a single physical characteristic. There are fat athletes, fat couch potatoes, fat people of every political and religious affiliation, disabled fat people, fat PhDs, fat queer people, fat people of color, and we go about the business of fighting our oppression in myriad ways. My goal with this anthology is to give you the opportunity to hear from and about as many of those people and types of activism as possible.

In a world where people ignore and ridicule actual fat people but clamor to hear about the experiences of celebrities in fat suits, and where government task forces are formed to "deal with the problem of obesity" without even one obese person included, where People of Size are talked about and talked at, but all too often not heard, I endeavored to take every opportunity to create a platform for People of Size to talk about our experiences. If you are a regular reader of anthologies, you'll definitely find pieces that are familiar to you, fully researched and written in the language of academia. You'll also find

first-person accounts of what it's like to be part of the Fat Acceptance movement. I've edited the pieces as little as possible to let the authors' voices shine
through, preferring to give readers a diverse collection of authentic voices and
working hard not to sacrifice that authenticity for consistency.

I encourage you to read with an open mind, and to remember that any feelings of disbelief or defensiveness are places to dig deeper, to check privilege,
and to remember that we are each the best witness to our own experiences,
welcome to ours.

1

Fat and Fit: Possible, Probable, Protective?

Angela Meadows

In his 1994 book *The Death of Humane Medicine and the Rise of Coercive Healthism*, Petr Skrabanek suggested that "healthism," the framing of the pursuit of health as a moral obligation, fills a void left by declining levels of religious belief in Western society and provides an alternative route to "salvation." Engagement in a "healthy lifestyle" results in avoidance of disease: those who participate, the righteous, will be rewarded; those who do not, the sinners, will be punished with ill health and untimely death.[1] In modern Western society, fat people have taken on the role of sinner. Guilty, apparently, of gluttony and sloth—two of the seven deadly sins—their fat bodies present a readily identifiable target for disapprobation, one that affords the virtuous an opportunity to shake their heads and rain down judgment on such scandalous eschewal of both individual and collective responsibility, reinforcing their own sense of moral superiority.

It is indeed possible that some fat people are guilty of these "vices," being both greedy and lazy. This is equally true for thin people. Others are not. While a critical analysis of healthism is beyond the scope of this chapter, I would like to address the misconception that all fat individuals spend their days sat on the sofa eating cheeseburgers. In particular, I will consider the case of exercise.

Contrary to popular belief, many fat people do engage in regular physical activity. Some are casual exercisers, some hike, some belly dance, some are more hard core—running marathons and taking part in extreme multiday endurance events—some are exercise instructors who teach daily aerobic classes, and some are semiprofessional or professional athletes.[2] I'm not describing individuals with high Body Mass Index (BMI)[3] due to increased muscularity—although fat people will have more muscle tissue, developed simply as a result of moving around a larger body—but rather people who exercise regularly and are still FAT.

The stereotype that fat people are inevitably idle arises, in part, from the widely held belief that exercise is a reliable means of achieving slimness. If this were indeed true, fat bodies, by their very existence, would represent visual proof of inactivity. However, modern research has consistently documented the limited response of body weight to physical activity. Weight loss results achieved in randomized controlled trials (the gold standard in research methods) of exercise interventions are generally poor, often in the range of only 2–3 kg (4.4–6.6 pounds) and less than one BMI unit over the course of a year.[4] This has been shown even in trials where regular, moderate to intense exercise was supervised, ruling out the possibility that people were not being truthful about how much activity they were doing.[5] A 2006 systematic review and meta-analysis looked at the results of 15 such trials that tested whether diet plus exercise resulted in more weight loss than diet alone; overall, the addition of exercise contributed only a 0.65 kg (1.4 pounds) greater weight loss, or less than one and a half pounds.[6] A 2009 review identified 18 randomized controlled trials of at least six months' duration that compared diet with diet plus exercise in adults. Eleven of these studies, comprising a total of 861 participants, measured weight loss in kilograms. They found that, overall, weight loss in the diet-only groups at the end of study follow-up was a not particularly earth-shattering 1.8 kg (3.9 pounds). The addition of exercise did increase weight loss, but only to 3.6 kg (7.9 pounds).[7] In other words, exercise contributed less than 2 kg (4.4 pounds) additional weight loss, consistent with the findings in the studies of exercise alone. The other seven trials, with 775 participants between them, reported changes in BMI rather than weight loss, and the results were equally unimpressive.[8]

All told, it seems that physical activity is not a particularly effective method of shedding pounds. It's not hard to understand why. To lose one pound in weight, you'd need to create a deficit of 3,500 calories;[9] that is, you'd have to use 3,500 calories more than you take in. Even assuming that every single calorie you expended exercising was equal to a one-calorie equivalent of weight loss, a woman weighing 100 kg (220 pounds), for example, would have to engage in more than five hours of jogging, rowing, cycling, or swimming, or more than 11 hours of walking at a moderate pace to lose *one pound*. It's easy to see that the amount of physical activity that would be needed to promote significant weight loss is likely to be unrealistic for most people. But many health and fitness professionals gloss over the relatively low caloric benefit of exercise, believing it may discourage people from being active. As both public health messages and popular media continue to promote exercise for its weight loss benefits rather than for its general health benefits, many people remain unaware of the amount of exercise needed to expend a significant number of calories and become rapidly discouraged when their efforts don't result in rapid weight loss.

But the true picture is even bleaker than this. In real life, a simple dose-response relationship between exercise energy expenditure and weight loss is rarely observed—that is, expending 3,500 calories in exercise is unlikely to give you a one-pound weight loss. The human body is very finely tuned and engages in a range of strategies to preserve itself, and the energy it needs to function, by any means necessary. Your body doesn't know that you're trying to lose weight and it compensates for the increase in energy expenditure (physical activity) by producing chemical messengers that increase appetite, driving you to eat more.[10] If you manage to resist the urge to eat more and stay on your diet, the body's internal metabolic regulation—the rate at which internal cellular processes operate and thus the amount of energy needed to complete them—must adapt. In lay terms, this is known as "slowing down your metabolism."[11]

There are other reasons why calories expended in exercise may not translate into equivalent amounts of weight loss. For example, if you exercise regularly, you may develop additional muscle mass.[12] This means that while your body composition changes, and your overall percentage of fat mass may be reduced, you might not see your efforts reflected on the scales. Both type and intensity of exercise,[13] as well as age, gender, ethnicity, peri-workout nutrition, and a history of weight cycling (yo-yo dieting) may also impact on the response to exercise.[14] In addition, genes are increasingly being shown to play a part in how and why people respond differently to exercise.[15]

One example of how genetic variability can impact on response to exercise is found in the effect of the fat mass and obesity-associated (FTO) gene, which comes in two flavors (in scientific terms, it has two allelic variants): A and C. People who carry the double AA genotype are predisposed to develop higher body weights, increasing the risk of becoming "obese" by two-thirds.[16] And in a nice double whammy, a 2010 study found that when 481 previously sedentary individuals underwent a 20-week supervised endurance exercise program, those carrying the AA form of the gene also experience two-thirds less fat loss compared with the other participants.[17] So, a genetic predisposition toward fatness may involve a number of different pathways, including a reduced body-weight response to exercise. While the amount of variation in adiposity explained by this one gene is small, dozens of obesity-linkage genetic variants have now been identified,[18] and it's clear that individual responses to energy intake and expenditure are more complex than a simple "calories in/calories out" model would suggest.

In 2012, an Australian team published a study in which they explored possible reasons for the less than expected weight loss during diet-plus-exercise interventions. Specifically, they were interested in the extent to which changes in metabolic rate and the composition of weight loss, i.e., fat tissue or muscle, were to blame. In their small but rigorously conducted study,

16 "obese" men and women were put on a 600-calorie-per-day diet for 12 weeks and, on top of this, were required to complete four aerobic sessions and two resistance training sessions each week, under supervision.[19] Despite the severe caloric restriction and the high-intensity, high-frequency exercise regimen, participants lost less weight than expected, largely due to compensatory slowing of their resting metabolic rate. Given that fat people who have attempted to lose weight through diet and exercise and who report lower than expected weight loss are usually accused of lying about the extent to which they have complied with their program, the authors' conclusions are worth noting:

> Although lower-than-expected weight loss is often attributed to incomplete adherence to prescribed interventions, the influence of baseline calculation errors and metabolic downregulation should not be discounted.[20]

Despite the generally lackluster effects of exercise on weight, large numbers of fat individuals continue to engage in regular physical activity, for a variety of reasons, including simple enjoyment. Consequently, many fat people are indeed relatively fit. A 2010 study of a subset of 4,675 adults from the U.S. National Health and Nutrition Examination Survey (NHANES I) who had performed submaximal exercise tests reported that while the percentage of individuals with a high level of cardiorespiratory fitness[21] was greater in "normal-weight" than "overweight" or "obese" individuals, nevertheless, 87.5 percent and 80 percent of "overweight" and "obese" individuals, respectively, achieved a moderate to high level of fitness.[22] Because people with some medical conditions that might make exercise testing risky were excluded from this part of the study for safety reasons, it's likely that those excluded may have represented some of the least fit individuals, and so these figures may well overestimate the proportion of fit people within the population as a whole, and those percentages should be interpreted with caution. Even so, it is clearly possible to be both "fat and fit," and large numbers of fat individuals are. Likewise, it is possible to be "normal weight" and have a low level of fitness. I'll come back to this.

So if it's not by causing weight loss that exercise makes us healthier, how does it work? Well, there are probably numerous mechanisms by which physical activity changes the body to improve health, and we're still discovering these, but one important one is via its effect on cardiorespiratory fitness. Although cardiorespiratory fitness is influenced by age, gender, health status, and genetic factors, habitual physical activity level is the principal modifiable component, i.e., the one we have any control over. Regular exercise is associated with adaptations in the circulatory, respiratory, and muscular symptoms that lead to increased aerobic fitness. Increased cardiorespiratory fitness is associated with reduced morbidity and all-cause mortality in men and women, independent of age, ethnicity, adiposity, smoking status, alcohol intake, and health conditions such as hypertension and diabetes.[23] This effect has been shown over and over again in numerous prospective longitudinal studies: more physical activity is associated with better life expectancy.[24]

Increasing amounts of evidence also suggest that the effects of many of the diseases associated with "obesity" can be ameliorated by lifestyle changes even in the absence of weight loss and that "obese" individuals are able to improve their health while remaining "obese."[25] Well-designed randomized controlled trials have demonstrated that increasing physical activity is associated with improvements in biochemical markers of health, including blood pressure, cholesterol, and insulin sensitivity,[26] and that many of these changes occur relatively rapidly—prior to any effects of increased physical activity on weight status. In fact, the benefits are accrued even if people don't lose any weight and can even be seen in people who gain weight.[27]

Strikingly, moderate to high cardiorespiratory fitness offsets at least some of the increased risk typically associated with fatness. Large epidemiological studies using objective measurements of cardiorespiratory fitness frequently report that "overweight" or "obese" individuals with high fitness levels have better long-term outcomes than "normal-weight" but unfit individuals.[28] And encouragingly, a systematic review of prospective longitudinal studies found a clear dose-response relationship between fitness and morbidity and mortality, with the greatest benefits associated with relatively small improvements in fitness that moved individuals out of the "least-fit" group.[29] So if you're currently in the nowhere-near-fit category, you can see significant health improvements by just getting yourself moving. And if you do, you'll be glad to know that when researchers followed a group of people over time, they found that unfit individuals who became fit had a relative risk of all-cause mortality on a par with fit individuals who became unfit, and this risk was lower than for those individuals who have stayed unfit (although it was still higher than for those who were fit at baseline and remained so at follow-up).[30]

Even more surprisingly, perhaps, the relationship between "obesity" and its "related diseases" isn't actually that strong, although you wouldn't know that from the ever-increasing hysteria in both the science and the lay literature. While an enormous amount of epidemiological evidence does show an association between "obesity" and morbidity and mortality,[31] these studies tend not to control for a range of confounding variables—other things that might affect the results—including physical activity level, fitness, or a history of weight cycling (otherwise known as yo-yo dieting). What's more, when possible confounders *are* corrected for, the association between obesity and disease is often significantly reduced or eliminated,[32] meaning that it could be these other factors, rather than the weight itself, that are behind the health issues.

In light of the growing body of evidence that weight loss neither is necessary for improved health nor indeed is even conducive to reducing morbidity and mortality risk, a new movement has emerged promoting "Health at Every Size" (HAES).[33] The HAES paradigm simply states that if an individual chooses to improve his or her health, whatever his or her size, the most useful way of achieving this is to adopt healthy behaviors and that the use of body weight or BMI as a proxy for health is neither reliable nor useful. Scientific evidence supporting this stance continues to emerge. For example, a 2012 analysis of nearly 12,000 individuals from the NHANES III cohort found that lifestyle was more important than weight for long-term outcomes.[34] The authors considered four "healthy habits": getting five or more servings of fruit and vegetables daily, exercising for at least 30 minutes three times a week, drinking alcohol only in moderation, and not smoking. For people with an unhealthy lifestyle—no healthy habits—weight was indeed important, with heavier individuals facing a significantly increased risk of all-cause mortality (compared with a "normal-weight" individual who engaged in all four habits); but for each health behavior added to one's lifestyle, the hazard ratio for all-cause mortality was reduced. Including just one healthy habit into your lifestyle removed most of the differences in risk between the three weight groups. With three healthy habits, the risk for "overweight" and "obese" individuals fell below that of even a "normal-weight" individual who did not achieve any of the habits; adopting all four healthy habits resulted in optimal and identical long-term outcomes, *irrespective of weight*. The importance of lifestyle factors over weight for long-term health outcomes is supported by a recently published prospective cohort study of nearly 72,000 Swedish men and women between the ages of 45 and 83.[35] When followed up for an average of 13 years, people who ate five or more servings of fruit and vegetables daily had the same long-term survival rates whether they fell into the "normal-weight" or "overweight" categories.[36]

Although it is clearly possible to be both fat and fit, and this state of affairs confers many health advantages, it is true that not all fat people have a good level of cardiorespiratory fitness. As with thin people, some will engage in regular physical activity whereas others will be more sedentary, although some will manage to maintain adequate levels of fitness even in the absence of exercise—having been blessed with "good genes." Cross-sectional studies and national statistical data do tend to show an inverse relationship between BMI and both physical activity level[37] and cardiorespiratory fitness[38]—that is, as BMI increases, the less likely individuals are to exercise regularly or maintain adequate levels of fitness. It should be noted, however, that these findings are not probative of a causal link—that fat people are fat because they do not exercise—and a number of alternative explanations for this relation-ship are possible.

On a pragmatic level, a range of practicalities may make it more difficult for the larger body to engage in many forms of physical activity—from the absence of suitable clothing and equipment, to the lack of understanding of the biomechanics of larger bodies among exercise professionals—making many attempts unnecessarily uncomfortable or even painful and dissuading further participation.[39] In addition, many fat people have spent their lives repeatedly engaging in cycles of diet and exercise while attempting to lose weight. They may have forced themselves to endure high-intensity activities that they disliked for the purpose of burning more calories. Yet as noted above, exercise, in the amounts achievable by the average working individual, is unlikely to lead to significant weight loss. Thus exercise becomes penance for being fat, yet provides little, if any, return in the form of weight loss, and many fat individuals have come to hate the entire process. Televisual reality shows such as *The Biggest Loser* also foster the notion that exercise must be punitive, with participants frequently shown vomiting, crying, and sustaining overuse injuries but forced to continue regardless, usually amid a torrent of verbal abuse from the show's trainers. Recent studies have shown, not entirely surprisingly, that watching *The Biggest Loser* tends to worsen viewers' attitudes toward exercise[40] and may discourage individuals from engaging in physical activity.[41] As noted above, the greatest benefits of increased fitness are accrued in individuals who change from being sedentary to engaging in any physical activity. Thus the idea that extreme exertion is necessary in order to reap health benefits is neither true nor helpful.

But perhaps more importantly, many fat individuals may avoid participa-tion in formal, or even informal, exercise due to embarrassment.[42] Experience of weight stigma has been linked to avoidance of exercise[43] and to less frequent engagement in moderate or strenuous exercise.[44] What's more, experiential avoidance and weight self-stigma are significant predictors of health-related quality of life and mediate the relationship between BMI and health-related quality of life.[45] In addition, weight self-stigma is inversely related to the pleasure and postexercise energy levels reported by "obese," but not "nonobese," women.[46] Activities such as fitness classes may include instructors openly stigmatizing fat bodies and encouraging participants to work harder to alleviate or prevent such a fate befalling them. Even moderate, non-gym-based activities such as walking and cycling can be traumatic experi-ences for the fat individual. Although few quantitative data on the prevalence of actual antifat stigmatization while exercising in public are available in the peer-review literature, numerous anecdotal accounts are available of peo-ple having things thrown at them, being verbally insulted, or even mooed at,[47] for the sin of exercising in public while fat.[48] And the recent interest in weight stigma has produced a slew of research papers that suggest the most common forms of stigmatization occur in public places—shops, restaurants, on the street, and so on.[49] Sadly, abusive remarks from strangers, being pointed at and laughed at by groups of people, and having insults hurled out of passing cars while out walking in public are not rare occurrences.[50] In one study of more than 2,000 individuals, 10 percent even reported being physically assaulted because of their weight.[51] And despite the fact that around two-thirds of individuals in the United States are now classified as "overweight" or "obese" (with similar rates in other Western countries), the problem of weight stigma appears to be getting worse.[52] Thus even for those who have not directly experienced these types of interactions, the not unreasonable fear that they may be subject to this kind of behavior is a very real deterrent to exercising in public.[53] The Internet and social media present a new outlet for antifat attitudes, and photos or videos of fat people exercising attract hordes of "trolls," who post everything from the most obscene insults to death threats in response.[54] Both individuals and organizations have used pictures of fat people engaging in exercise as a highly derogatory source of humor.[55] Fat athletes are generally ignored or sidelined by the media, and attempts to show fat individuals engaging in healthy behaviors are often met with accusations that the source is "promoting obesity."[56] Thus fat individuals, of all ages, lack role models on whom they can base their own aspirations.

The aversion to showing exercising fat people in a positive light, or at all for that matter, has far-reaching and paradoxical implications.[57] Health psychology research has shown that Bandura's social cognitive theory[58] accounts for a significant proportion of the variance between individuals with respect to a range of health behaviors, including participation in physical activity.[59] The major determinant of social cognitive theory is self-efficacy, an individual's belief in his or her ability to successfully accomplish an activity, which has been shown to be one of the most robust psychosocial predictors of physical activity and exercise.[60] Interventions that lead to increased physical activity self-efficacy result in increased and more sustained participation in exercise.[61] Not seeing a single example of somebody who looks like you taking part in sports and other fitness activities will do nothing to foster self-efficacy and is likely to be associated with reduced participation among fat individuals.

Although exercise is unlikely to lead to weight loss in the majority of participants, there is a strong argument for public health messages to promote exercise and physical activity in their own right, for *all* people, not just the fat ones. Cross-sectional studies in both healthy and disease populations have found that increased physical activity level is associated with a range of physical, cognitive, and emotional improvements and with improved health-related quality of life.[62] But which comes first? It could be that happy, healthy people exercise more, or it could be that exercise makes people happy and healthy. In all likelihood, it's probably a virtuous circle in which both of these are true. But a recent randomized controlled trial conducted on 430 postmenopausal "overweight" and "obese" women (BMI 25.0–43.0) who were sedentary at the start of the study showed that both physical and mental aspects of health-related quality of life were improved with exercise in a dose-dependent manner.[63] In other words, the more people exercised, at least within the levels considered in this study (up to 150% of the National Institutes for Health guidelines for physical activity), the better their quality of life. That is, exercise makes people happy and healthy, or at least happier and healthier. The study also showed that these improvements in health occurred independent of weight loss.

The continued focus of public health efforts on the promotion of weight loss as a primary goal may be not only ineffective but also stigmatizing and unhelpful. In response to the difficulties and prejudiced faced by many fat exercises, the Fit Fatties Forum[64] was set up by two fat activists: Ragen Chastain, a dancer, choreographer, and writer; and Jeanette DePatie, a certified fitness instructor who teaches regular aerobic classes and runs marathons and triathlons in her spare time. Both of them are fat. The Fit Fatties Forum is a HAES-friendly space where people of all sizes and abilities with an interest in exercise can receive support, connect with others, and make friends, without a focus on weight loss.

The responses of many nonfat individuals to the existence of such a space is indicative of the harm engendered by the current weight-based paradigm. In her blog *Dances with Fat*, Ms. Chastain has cataloged some of the more printable responses she receives when publicizing the Fit Fatties Forum. The following is a typical example that highlights the extent of the problem:

> I looked at your fat people forum—I think you people need to stop running marathons and start focusing on losing weight.[65]

Further, from a public health perspective, weight-based messages may miss a significant proportion of the "normal-weight" population who are at increased risk of ill health due to their lifestyles, while targeting a proportion of the "overweight and obese" population who are not. Increasing engagement in exercise and physical activity would be a more useful target for public health policies and interventions. Weight loss may or may not be a by-product of such activities but is not a necessary prerequisite for individuals to achieve the health benefits associated with physical activity, including higher fitness levels, better metabolic health, greater self-efficacy, improved mood, and higher health-related quality of life.

In a 2009 review entitled "The Future of Obesity Reduction: Beyond Weight Loss," Ross and Bradshaw stated:

A preoccupation with weight loss as the primary determinant of success-ful obesity reduction is not supported from either a biological or behav-ioral perspective. ... Little support exists for the position that weight loss is an absolute requirement if obese individuals are to experience a health benefit, or that a weight reduction of ≥5% is a threshold that must be achieved to reduce obesity-related risks to health. On the con-trary, several lines of evidence underscore the health benefits of lifestyle-based strategies that include an increase in physical activity combined with a healthy diet, independent of changes in weight.[66]

The move away from a focus on weight loss as a means to achieve health is gaining traction among many researchers and clinicians, yet its assimilation into the mainstream has been slow, possibly due to powerful vested financial and professional interests. Yet the current "obesity epidemic" hysteria is help-ing nobody, of any weight. It is time for a paradigm shift. Until our govern-ments and our medical professionals take on this message, we alone can advocate for and champion our own health agendas.

Despite current public health messages that fat people need to engage in exer-cise, automatically assuming that they currently do not, society at large is not kind to the fat exerciser. If public health messages are indeed intended to improve the health of the public, a more useful approach should be to work to reduce the stigma so ingrained in our society and to promote physical activity for *all* bodies. People of all shapes and sizes will profit from the numerous benefits that physical activity can bring, not just in terms of fitness and improved physical health but also in improved psychosocial well-being, occasions shared with friends and colleagues, immersion in nature, and the like. One of the many casu-alties of the current "war on obesity" is that we appear to have forgotten how to move our bodies for the sheer enjoyment of it. This needs to change.

Finally, as the modern-day versions of gluttony and sloth—eating fast food and abstaining from circuit classes, either in actuality or perceived—appear to have become a measure of human decency and worth, it might behoove us to remember that pride, or hubris—the desire, among other things, to be more important or attractive than others—has throughout history been considered the most serious of the deadly sins.

NOTES

1. Petr Skrabanek, *The Death of Humane Medicine and the Rise of Coercive Healthism* (London: Social Affairs Unit, 1994), 17.

2. Candice Buss, "Social Networking and the Fat Female Athlete: Reimagining the Female Athlete" (presentation, annual meeting of the National Women's Studies Association, Atlanta, GA, November 29, 2011).

3. Body mass index (BMI) is a measure of bodily stature, calculated as weight in kilograms divided by height in meters squared (or weight in pounds times 703 divided by height in inches squared). In 1998, the World Health Organization designated cutoffs for "underweight" (BMI less than 18.5), "normal weight" (BMI 18.5–24.9), "overweight" (BMI 25–29.9), and "obese" (BMI over 30). World Health Organization, "Obesity: Preventing and Managing the Global Epdiemic," Report of a WHO Consultation on Obesity (Geneva: World Health Organization, 1998). These categories are widely used in scientific studies of weight and health and will be adopted here when they refer to specific research conducted based on these criteria.

4. K. Shaw et al., "Exercise for Overweight or Obesity," *Cochrane Database of Systematic Reviews* 4 (2006): 56.

5. Ibid. Four included studies had interventions involving supervised exercise: Jeffery (1998), Neumark (1995), Stefanik (1998), and Svendsen (1993).

6. Ibid., 58.

7. T. Wu et al., "Long-Term Effectiveness of Diet-Plus-Exercise Interventions vs. Diet-Only Interventions for Weight Loss: A Meta-Analysis," *Obesity Reviews* 10, no. 3 (2009): 319.

8. Ibid.

9. Technically, this should be "kilocalories," but I will use the widely accepted lay version of this term, "calorie," in this chapter.

10. Priya Sumithran and Joseph Proietto, "The Defence of Body Weight: A Physiological Basis for Weight Regain after Weight Loss," *Clinical Science* 124 (2013): 234–35.

11. M. Rosenbaum and R. L. Leibel, "Adaptive Thermogenesis in Humans," *International Journal of Obesity* 34 (2010): S48; Sumithran and Proietto, "The Defence of Body Weight," 232–33.

12. D. L. Ballor and E. T. Poehlman, "Exercise-Training Enhances Fat-Free Mass Preservation during Diet-Induced Weight Loss: A Meta-Analytical Finding," *International Journal of Obesity and Related Metabolic Disorders* 18, no. 1 (1994): 35.

13. G. R. Hunter et al., "A Role for High Intensity Exercise on Energy Balance and Weight Control," *International Journal of Obesity and Related Metabolic Disorders* 22, no. 6 (1998): 489.

14. S. H. Boutcher and S. L. Dunn, "Factors That May Impede the Weight Loss Response to Exercise-Based Interventions," *Obesity Reviews* 10, no. 6 (2009): 676.

15. Tuomo Rankinen and Claude Bouchard, "Gene-Physical Activity Interactions: Overview of Human Studies," *Obesity (Silver Spring)* 16, suppl. 3 (2008): S47.

16. R. J. Loos and C. Bouchard, "FTO: The First Gene Contributing to Common Forms of Human Obesity," *Obesity Reviews* 9, no. 3 (2008): 246.

17. Tuomo Rankinen et al., "FTO Genotype Is Associated with Exercise Training-Induced Changes in Body Composition," *Obesity (Silver Springs)* 18, no. 2 (2010): 325.

18. Felix R. Day and Ruth J. F. Loos, "Developments in Obesity Genetics in the Era of Genome-Wide Association Studies," *Journal of Nutrigenetics and Nutrigenomics* 4, no. 4 (2011): 222.

19. N. M. Byrne et al., "Does Metabolic Compensation Explain the Majority of Less-Than-Expected Weight Loss in Obese Adults during a Short-Term Severe Diet and Exercise Intervention?," *International Journal of Obesity* 36, no. 11 (2012): 1473.

20. Ibid.,1478.

21. Cardiorespiratory fitness (or aerobic fitness) is a measure of the body's ability to respond to physical demand by delivering sufficient oxygen to metabolically active tissues to support sustained physical activity. Duck-chul Lee et al., "Mortality Trends in the General Population: The Importance of Cardiorespiratory Fitness," *Journal of Psychopharmacology* 24, suppl. 4 (2010).

22. Glen E. Duncan, "The 'Fit but Fat' Concept Revisited: Population-Based Estimates Using NHANES," *International Journal of Behavioral Nutrition and Physical Activity* 7 (2010): 4.

23. Lee et al., "Mortality Trends in the General Population," 28.

24. James Woodcock et al., "Non-Vigorous Physical Activity and All-Cause Mortality: Systematic Review and Meta-Analysis of Cohort Studies," *International Journal of Epidemiology* 40, no. 1 (2011): 121.

25. Linda Bacon and Lucy Aphramor, "Weight Science: Evaluating the Evidence for a Paradigm Shift," *Nutrition Journal* 10 (2011): 2.

26. Shaw et al., "Exercise for Overweight or Obesity," 1.

27. Bacon and Aphramor, "Weight Science," 6.

28. Lee et al., "Mortality Trends in the General Population," 28.

29. Woodcock et al., "Non-Vigorous Physical Activity," 121.

30. Lee et al., "Mortality Trends in the General Population," 29.

31. Katherine M. Flegal et al., "Cause-Specific Excess Deaths Associated with Underweight, Overweight, and Obesity," *Journal of the American Medical Association* 298, no. 1 (2005): 2031.

32. Paul Campos et al., "The Epidemiology of Overweight and Obesity: Public Health Crisis or Moral Panic?," *International Journal of Epidemiology* 35, no. 1 (2006): 56.

33. Bacon and Aphramor, "Weight Science," 8.

34. Eric M. Matheson, Dana E. King, and Charles J. Everett, "Healthy Lifestyle Habits and Mortality in Overweight and Obese Individuals," *Journal of the American Board of Family Medicine* 25, no. 1 (2012): 13.

35. Andrea Bellavia et al., "Fruit and Vegetable Consumption and All-Cause Mortality: A Dose-Response Analysis," *American Journal of Clinical Nutrition* 98, no. 2 (2013): 454.

36. Andrea Bellavia, e-mail message to author, November 29, 2013.

37. Centers for Disease Control and Prevention, *Adult Participation in Aerobic and Muscle-Strengthening Physical Activities—United States, 2011*, Morbidity and Mortality Weekly Report, no. 62, May 3, 2013, http://www.cdc.gov/mmwr/preview/mmwrhtml/mm6217a2.htm?s_cid=mm6217a2_w.

38. Susan G. Lakoski et al., "Impact of Body Mass Index, Physical Activity, and Other Clinical Factors on Cardiorespiratory Fitness (from the Cooper Center Longitudinal Study)," *American Journal of Cardiology* 108, no. 1 (2011): 37.

39. Jaclyn Packer, "The Role of Stigmatization in Fat People's Avoidance of Physical Exercise," *Women & Therapy* 8, no. 3 (1989): 56–57.

40. Tanya R. Berry et al., "Effects of Biggest Loser Exercise Depictions on Exercise-Related Attitudes," *American Journal of Health Behavior* 37, no. 1 (2013): 100.

41. Tucker Readdy and Vicki Ebbeck, "Weighing In on NBC's The Biggest Loser," *Research Quarterly for Exercise and Sport* 83, no. 4 (2013): 584.

42. Sophie Lewis et al., "How Do Obese Individuals Perceive and Respond to the Different Types of Obesity Stigma That They Encounter in Their Daily Lives? A Qualitative Study," *Social Science & Medicine* 73, no. 9 (2011): 1354.

43. Dorothy L. Schmalz, " 'I Feel Fat': Weight-Related Stigma, Body Esteem, and BMI as Predictors of Perceived Competence in Physical Activity," *Obesity Facts* 3, no. 1 (2010): 18; Lenny R. Vartanian and Jacqueline G. Shaprow, "Effects of Weight Stigma on Exercise Motivation and Behavior: A Preliminary Investigation among College-Aged Females," *Journal of Health Psychology* 13, no. 1 (2008): 131.

44. Ibid.

45. Jason Lillis, Michael E. Levin, and Steven Hayes, "Exploring the Relationship between BMI and Health-Related Quality of Life: A Pilot Study of the Impact of Weight Self-Stigma and Experiential Avoidance," *Journal of Health Psychology* 16, no. 5 (2011): 1.

46. Panteleimon Ekkekakis, Erik Lind, and Spiridoula Vazou, "Affective Responses to Increasing Levels of Exercise Intensity in Normal-Weight, Overweight, and Obese Middle-Aged Women," *Obesity (Silver Spring)* 18, no. 1 (2010): 79.

47. While researching this chapter, I even came across a Facebook page with the charming name "Yelling 'Moo' at fat people." Hopefully, following complaints to Facebook administrators, this page will no longer exist at time of going to press.

48. Jean Braithwaite, "Fat Pride," *Sun*, no. 379, July 2007, http://thesunmagazine. org/issues/379/fat_pride; Ragen *Chastain*, "To the Guys Who Threw Eggs at Me Tonight," *Dances with Fat* (blog), August 23, 2013, http://danceswithfat.wordpress. com/2013/08/23/to-the-guys-who-threw-eggs-at-me-tonight/; Vivian F. Mayer, "The Fat Illusion," in *Shadow on a Tightrope: Writings by Women on Fat Oppression*, ed. Lisa Schoenenfielder and Barb Wieser (Iowa City: Aunt Lute Book Company, 1983), 8; Lonie McMichael, *Acceptable Prejudice? Fat, Rhetoric and Social Justice* (Nashville, TN: Pearlsong Press, 2013), 34.

49. Deborah Carr and Michael A. Friedman, "Is Obesity Stigmatizing? Body Weight, Perceived Discrimination, and Psychological Well-Being in the United States," *Journal of Health and Social Behavior* 46, no. 3 (2005): 251; Mark L. Hatzenbuehler, Katherine M. Keyes, and Deborah S. Hasin, "Associations between Perceived Weight Discrimination and the Prevalence of Psychiatric Disorders in the General Population," *Obesity* 17, no. 11 (2009): 2036; R. M. Puhl, T. Andreyeva, and K. D. Brownell, "Perceptions of Weight Discrimination: Prevalence and Comparison to Race and Gender Discrimination in America," *International Journal of Obesity* 14, no. 10 (2006): 997.

50. Puhl, Andreyeva and Brownell, 1806, 1808. The measure used in this study was the Stigmatizing Situations Inventory (Myers and Rosen 1999). It comprises

11 situational subscales, including health care, comments from children, family, being stared at, and receiving nasty comments from others (friends, strangers, etc.). Items include "Groups of people pointing and laughing at you in public," "When walking outside, having people drive by and laugh or shout insults," and "Being hit, beaten up, or physically attacked because of your weight."

51. Ibid.

52. Tatiana Andreyeva, Rebecca M. Puhl, and Kelly D. Brownell, "Changes in Perceived Weight Discrimination among Americans, 1995–1996 through 2004–2006," *Obesity* 16, no. 5 (2008): 1132.

53. Lewis et al., "How Do Obese Individuals Perceive," 1352.

54. Lonie McMichael, *Talking Fat: Health vs. Persuasion in the War on Our Bodies* (Nashville, TN: Pearlsong Press, 2012), 12; McMichael, *Acceptable Prejudice?*, 78.

55. Ragen Chastain, "Miami City Ballet and What Not to Do," *Dances with Fat* (blog), November 25, 2012, http://danceswithfat.wordpress.com/2012/11/25/miami-city-ballet-and-what-not-to-do/.

56. Ragen Chastain, "The 'Promoting Obesity' Myth," *Dances with Fat* (blog), December 9, 2011, http://danceswithfat.wordpress.com/2011/12/09/the-promoting-obesity-myth/.

57. Lewis et al., "How Do Obese Individuals Perceive," 1353.

58. Albert Bandura, *Self-Efficacy: The Exercise of Control* (New York: Freeman, 1997).

59. Barbara Resnick et al., "Path Analysis of Efficacy Expectations and Exercise Behaviour in Older Adults," *Journal of Advanced Nursing* 31, no. 6 (2000): 1309.

60. Adrian E. Bauman et al., "Correlates of Physical Activity: Why Are Some People Physically Active and Others Not?," *Lancet* 380, no. 9838 (2012) : 260.

61. S. L. Williams and D. P. French, "What Are the Most Effective Intervention Techniques for Changing Physical Activity Self-Efficacy and Physical Activity Behaviour—and Are They the Same?" *Health Education Research* 26, no. 2 (2011): 312.

62. Raphaël Bize, Jeffrey A. Johnson, and Ronald C. Plotnikoff, "Physical Activity Level and Health-Related Quality of Life in the General Adult Population: A Systematic Review," *Preventive Medicine* 45, no. 6 (2007): 409.

63. Corby K. Martin et al., "Exercise Dose and Quality of Life: A Randomized Controlled Trial," *Archives of Internal Medicine* 169, no. 3 (2009): 269.

64. Fitfatties.ning.com.

65. Ragen Chastain, "Holy Mixed Messages Fatman," *Dances with Fat* (blog), December 15, 2012, http://danceswithfat.wordpress.com/2012/12/15/holy-mixed-messages-fatman/.

66. Robert Ross and Alison J. Bradshaw, "The Future of Obesity Reduction: Beyond Weight Loss," *Nature Reviews Endocrinology* 5, no. 6 (2009): 319–20.

2

New Frontiers in Weight Bias: The Womb as Ground Zero in the War on Obesity

Pamela Vireday

Not satisfied with their lack of progress in eradicating obesity in society, public health advocates have now moved the battle onto a new field of combat—the wombs of the world. They are intent on wiping out obesity before it even begins by targeting fat women who might reproduce.

In order to do this, they have:

- Instituted a media campaign to discourage as many women of size from pregnancy as possible
- Made health care providers the gatekeepers of reproduction in order to bully women into losing weight before pregnancy or fertility treatment
- Institutionalized weight bias by ghettoizing fat women into "bariatric obstetrics" clinics that make high-intervention birth and fat shaming the norm
- Targeted obesity in the womb by putting the baby on a diet before it is even born

Of course, it's important to note that not all providers are unsupportive of fat women during pregnancy. Some are relatively weight-neutral and provide reasonable care. Some provide truly gentle, respectful care for women of size. Some gems actively advocate for better treatment of fat women and challenge the weight bias that is so rampant in the obstetric world.

But when you look at the public health messages, the practices of many care providers, and the experiences of fat women, it is obvious that there is definitely an insidious campaign toward eradicating obesity at its earliest possible stages, either by discouraging reproduction in fat women in the first place or by imposing draconian protocols on fat women around pregnancy.

The rhetoric around obesity and pregnancy has reached new, increasingly sensationalistic levels in recent years. Articles strongly emphasize the risks, highlight supersized women as if they represent the majority of obese women, rarely portray positive outcomes, and call for women to lose weight before pregnancy, despite the lack of effective programs that provide sustainable weight loss.[1] Look at the alarming headlines from a few recent articles:

- The #1 Pregnancy Risk[2]
- 10 Scary Reasons to Fight Obesity Before Pregnancy[3]
- Fat Mothers Putting Babies' Health at Risk[4]
- Pregnancy & Obesity: A Dangerous Combo[5]

Articles like these play up risk and use frightening, attention-grabbing language like "dangerous," "ticking time bomb," "runaway train," and other, similar phrases.[6] One opinion piece states:

> Obesity creates a murderers' row of obstetrical miseries . . . Deliveries are messy and dangerous. There's the anecdote of a baby who almost drowned in the wall of fat of a severely overweight c-section patient . . . Studies of women who were obese before pregnancy, or gained too much weight during pregnancy, reveal a whole grab-bag of fetal development horrors.[7]

These articles rarely place the risks they discuss in context or give actual numerical estimations associated with these risks.[8] If they did, readers would see that, although at increased risk for some things,[9] *most* fat women do not experience the given particular complication.[10] After reading some of these articles, one would think that *no* fat pregnant woman has ever had a healthy pregnancy or a healthy baby.[11]

Images in these stories often feature "headless fatties" who are sedentary, eating unhealthy foods, shot from unflattering angles, or wearing very tight clothes.[12] These pictures are very stigmatizing and have a negative influence on viewers' perception of fat people.[13] In this way, they help shape public condemnation around obesity and pregnancy.

Often these articles tell an apocryphal story of an obese woman with severe complications, implying that all fat women are at equal risk for such a dire outcome.[14] Or they discuss women of the highest weights, as if this is representative of the experiences of most fat women.[15] They particularly love to tell the story of a fat woman who ate poorly but who now has been shown "the error of her ways."[16]

The clear message is condemnation and pressure to lose weight. Fat women are foolishly endangering their babies by daring to even consider pregnancy while obese, and any fat woman who gets pregnant without losing weight first is the "ultimate bad mother."[17] As one blogger put it, "Fat is the new crack" in bad-mother blaming.[18]

There is a special sense of moral panic and blaming around messages about the "obesity epidemic."[19] This is even stronger in the messages around fatness and pregnancy. If you look closely, there is more than a tinge of racism and classism in rhetoric of these stories,[20] as there often is when discussing the "obesity epidemic."[21] The fat mothers featured in these cautionary tales are often women of color, and the neighborhoods targeted for special "obesity in pregnancy" clinics are often neighborhoods of poor minority women.[22]

Sexism, too, is strong in these messages. One author notes, "Requirements of self-regulation regarding weight during pregnancy hold women individually responsible for any future deviations of the 'normal' weight of their child."[23] In other words, the pregnant woman's actions regarding her weight before and during pregnancy mean that she is responsible for her child's health and his or her weight trajectory *forever*. This is mother guilting taken to a new level.

Messages discouraging pregnancy in women of size don't have to be overt to be influential. Pregnant women of size are invisible except as targets of negative media coverage. The lack of pictures of fat women in pregnancy and breastfeeding resources, the lack of plus sizes in many maternity stores, and the dearth of positive birth stories of women of size all portray a clear message—Thou Shalt Not Reproduce.

The next step in taking the war on obesity to the womb is to make care providers the gatekeepers of the right to procreate.

Care providers have been convinced by media campaigns that pregnancy at larger sizes is *far* too dangerous, and they do whatever it takes to keep fat women from having babies. That may involve medical bullying by scaring fat women from pregnancy, strong-arming them into drastic weight loss, encouraging termination of pregnancies, or forbidding fertility treatments.

The first step is well on its way. Many doctors have become "scare providers" instead of "care providers."[24] Instead of a reasoned dialogue about the possible risks of pregnancy at larger sizes, discussions about risk are often turned into patronizing and fat-shaming lectures. Disaster scenarios and worst possible outcomes are emphasized in an effort to scare women out of considering pregnancy:[25]

Obese women are more likely to have miscarriages and malformed babies and 50 per cent of them will have to give birth by caesarean section—often weeks before the child is due ... large babies born to obese women often had their shoulders stuck in the birth canal and this could lower the baby's oxygen levels and leave them with injuries or nerve problems.

It's not that possible risks of obesity and pregnancy shouldn't be discussed with clients; women deserve to be informed of the possible risks.[26] However, it needs to be done in a fair and balanced way, giving women actual numerical incidence of complications rather than ominous pronouncements of increased risk.[27] Furthermore, the risks need to be presented in a nonjudgmental and undistorted way, acknowledging that many women of size actually do have healthy pregnancies and babies.[28]

Unfortunately, many practitioners have developed such an exaggerated sense of risk around pregnancy in high-weight women that they no longer see the potential for complications but rather the *certainty* of them. Some women are even told that they probably won't survive the pregnancy:[29]

- If you get pregnant, you will get gestational diabetes, have high blood pressure, and oh, you will probably just die anyway.
- [My doctor] basically made me feel my baby is a death sentence . . . In his "honest opinion" I am going to die during labor/delivery or recovery.
- [The doctor] told me that I wasn't going to make it alive through my pregnancy . . . he kept saying I shouldn't have gotten pregnant, that I had in a sense, committed suicide.
- If you labor, you'll have a heart attack and die on the table.

Some fat women are told that their baby will be born unhealthy or would be unlikely to survive the pregnancy:[30]

- Because you are obese, you will have a deformed baby.
- [My doctor] said that "at your age and with your size" that either the baby or I would die.
- The baby would only have a 5% chance of survival.

Some mothers are even encouraged to terminate the pregnancy:[31]

- [The doctor] spoke on and on about why it probably wasn't a good idea for me to have the baby and that time was running short for me to terminate the pregnancy.
- When I got pregnant I was told by various doctors for various reasons that I should abort.
- I spent hours on the phone looking for a doctor that wouldn't counsel immediate termination ("You or the baby will die, you are just too fat to carry to term").

Other women of size are pressured to have their tubes tied at birth to prevent further pregnancies.[32] Even in adoption, fat women are often prevented from becoming parents.[33] The official position of the American Congress of Obstetricians and Gynecologists is that obese women should be encouraged "to undertake a weight-reduction program" before pregnancy.[34] Some care providers don't stop there; they imply that the *only* way to have a healthy baby is to lose weight first.[35] Women are repeatedly told in the media that they are putting their health at risk and face greater risks of illness and death if they don't lose substantial amounts of weight before pregnancy.[26]

Although there is research showing some benefits to weight reduction before or between pregnancies,[37] there is also research to suggest that dieting or weight reduction near the time of conception is associated with higher risks for birth defects.[38] Obese women who lose weight between pregnancies or who are chronic dieters also often have greater weight gain in the next pregnancy,[39] which may also be harmful.[40]

In addition, the failure rate among dieters is very high.[41] If studied long enough, most people regain the lost weight[42] and often end up at a higher weight than they started.[43] Even among people who lose weight long term, few are able to reduce their weight into "normal" body mass index (BMI) ranges.[44] And dieting before pregnancy puts the woman at risk for nutritional shortfalls, just when nutritional demands are at their peak.[45]

Thus delaying pregnancy until weight is "normalized" may keep fat women from *ever* having a baby. Fat women who want a family have to weigh possible advantages of delaying pregnancy until weight is normalized against the decrease in fertility and increased risk for complications associated with pregnancy at older ages. Some fat women have opted for emphasizing healthy behaviors over losing weight before pregnancy, yet many providers see only an either/or choice—lose weight or don't get pregnant.

Because of their extreme perception of risk in obese women, many doctors feel justified in denying fat women fertility help.[46] Many women of size report that they have been denied fertility treatment unless they lost weight first:[47]

- I was refused fertility treatment on the NHS [National Health Service, United Kingdom] in 2008 due to my BMI being above 30 ... When we went to a private clinic we found that the BMI restrictions apply everywhere, not just on the NHS.
- I went to the [reproductive endocrinologist] for infertility. She refused to treat me because of my weight ... I have perfect blood pressure, cholesterol, and I am not diabetic. I am married, financially stable, and a productive member of society. Why don't I deserve the chance to be a mother?
- [The doctor said,] "Fat women only have babies because we can't stop them, we're certainly not going to help you conceive."

They cite reasons like limited funding, lower rates of successful treatment, and an increased risk for pregnancy complications in obese women.[48] Yet women over 35 have higher costs, lower success rates, and higher complication rates, but that does not automatically exclude them from fertility treatment.[49] Why should obesity be different?

Some infertility specialists tell fat women that because they are at increased risk for complications in pregnancy, it would be unethical to help them achieve pregnancy. Some even call it "tantamount to child abuse."[50] Dr. Arthur Leader of the Ottawa Fertility Centre, who opposes fertility treatment for morbidly obese women, said, "A patient doesn't have the right to make a choice that's going to be harmful to them."[51]

Many other groups of women are at risk for complications in pregnancy, like those with type 1 diabetes, blood-clotting disorders, or lupus. Yet these women receive treatment in many fertility clinics.[52] The difference is that these women are seen as being victims of genetic bad luck, whereas obesity is viewed as a voluntary condition, caused by poor lifestyle, ignorance, or weak willpower.[53] The bottom line is that many infertility doctors don't believe that fat women *deserve* to have babies because they see fat women as stubbornly refusing to "get healthy."

Many women of size actually have a condition called polycystic ovarian syndrome (PCOS), a hormonal disorder that interferes with ovulation and that often makes it difficult to lose weight. In denying fat women with PCOS access to fertility treatments, are they discriminating against the very women who need the treatment the most? While doctors like to pretend that access to fertility treatment is about economics and risk mitigation, what's really at the heart of it is weight bias.

History shows that marginalized groups are often discouraged from reproducing, sometimes by force. Scaring fat women out of pregnancy, pressuring them for abortion, requiring radical weight loss, or denying them fertility treatment has the same effect as forced sterilization in the end. The war on obesity in the womb is just the latest version of the eugenics movement.

Another response to obesity and pregnancy concerns has been to call for specialized centers for treating fat women.[54] This can sound good on paper— size-appropriate equipment and additional resources in case of severe complications—but it can also backfire by forcing fat women into a high-intervention model of care and very strong pressure for women to diet aggressively postpartum.[55]

Because of the push for bariatric obstetric practices, some women of size— even ones with no complications—are being turned away from regular providers and sent to high-risk specialists.[56] Others are being told they cannot birth in a local hospitals but must go to regional hospitals instead.[57]

Pregnant women of size don't want to be sent to fat gulags where strong-arm tactics are the norm. Forcing obese women into high-intervention care models is a violation of the right to patient autonomy. To paraphrase Susan Hodges of *Citizens for Midwifery*, "How much perceived 'risk' does it take to supersede a mother's right to patient autonomy?" Fat women should be able to birth where and with whom they choose.

Given the highly profitable weight loss industry, hard questions must also be asked about the profit motive of this movement toward specialist clinics. Bariatric obstetrics is potentially a very lucrative business model. It utilizes expensive high-risk consultants for routine care, whether or not fat women actually experience complications. And it often incorporates costly tests and consults, not to mention "bariatricians" who design specialized plans for obese women to "reeducate" them about healthy eating.[58]

The attitude toward women of size in these clinics is often patronizing and condescending.[59] Weight stigma is already a serious problem in maternity care.[60] Will bariatric obstetric clinics help the problem or just exacerbate it further?

Another problem with bariatric obstetrics is that it ghettoizes obese women into high-intervention care, which is associated with extremely high cesarean rates.[61] The cesarean rate is already nearly 50 percent in "morbidly obese" women in some studies and can reach as high as 70 percent.[62] This is a concern because cesareans carry increased risks for complications in women of size, including infections, anesthetic problems, blood clots, and wound complications.[63] In addition, every successive cesarean increases the risk for complications in future pregnancies, including placental issues, hemorrhage, and hysterectomy.[64]

Reducing the high cesarean rate in women of size is a critical issue in improving outcomes in this group. There is good reason to believe that cesarean rates can be reduced by keeping low-intervention care available, avoiding unnecessary planned cesareans, lowering induction rates, and avoiding obstetric interventions whenever possible.

Research is clear that midwifery and low-intervention care can lower the risk for cesareans for women in general.[65] Even in women with "moderate" risk factors, a low-intervention model of care had equivalent or better outcomes.[66] Yet the increased emphasis on specialized bariatric obstetric centers decreases fat women's ability to choose midwifery and low-tech care, denying them a powerful tool for lowering their risk for surgery:[67]

- [The midwife] informed me that this group does not accept patients with a BMI over 40.
- I went to a birthing center and they told me that they only take patients with BMIs up to 40.

- Because of your weight, you're just not a candidate for midwifery care, and we're going to go ahead and get you to an OB to schedule your cesarean section.

Another problem is the common obstetric belief that fat women can't or shouldn't give birth vaginally. Increasingly, many providers just schedule high-BMI women for a cesarean preemptively:[68]

- I was told during my second pregnancy... that I would have to have a c-section because I am fat ... I ended up having a straightforward natural (2 hour) labour and delivery.
- Women of your size never have a natural labor. You will have to have a c-section.
- When an anonymous survey was conducted, 100% of the OBs at this hospital ... admitted that they would schedule a c-section automatically if a woman's BMI was over 30 and there were any other risk factors, or BMI over 40 with no other problems.

Planned c-sections without labor in high-BMI patients continue to be routine in many areas, yet research shows that many morbidly obese women can birth vaginally if given adequate opportunity:[69]

[This study] challenge[s] the assumption that elective CS [cesarean section or c-section] is safer than planned vaginal delivery in these morbidly obese women. A large proportion, 70% of women with BMI $\geq$ 50 kd/m2 ... did indeed delivery vaginally without the expected increase in neonatal and postnatal complication rates compared with those with planned elective CS. These data strongly indicate that elective CS in morbidly obese women cannot be justified.[70]

Yet even when allowed to labor, women of size are often managed straight into cesareans by being required to have additional interventions, such as induction of labor, being confined to bed, early placement of an epidural, breaking the waters early, and aggressive augmentation drugs.[71]

The factor with the most impact is the high induction rate, which is common even when no complications are present.[72] In some studies, 50 to 60 percent of morbidly obese women were induced,[73] even though induced labor increases the risk for cesareans.[74] The authors of one study found, "A morbidly obese woman in spontaneous labour has a 70% chance of achieving a vaginal delivery but this falls to only 48% if labour is induced."[75]

Yet most researchers still fail to connect the dots between high induction rates and high cesarean rates in obese women.[76]

Research suggests that a difference in labor management can result in strikingly different outcomes. In one Kentucky study, for example, the cesarean rate was nearly 60 percent in women with a BMI $\geq$ 50, yet a British study of similarly sized women found a cesarean rate of only 30 percent.[77] More study is needed, but individualizing care and keeping low-intervention care models available may be the key to helping high-weight women have the best chance at a normal, nonsurgical birth.[78]

As you might expect, interference in bariatric obstetrics doesn't end with birth. Afterward, women often face extreme pressure to lose weight. Providers use emotionally loaded arguments to manipulate women into dieting postpartum, such as:[79]

- [My doctor] . . . told me that I couldn't even consider the idea of having another baby or I would die for sure.
- If I did not [diet], I would be dead before ten years, because women my size don't live past 40.
- [Your] child will never love [you] because he would be so ashamed to have a fat mama.

This type of medical bullying may backfire. Stigmatizing words and practices do not improve outcome and may actually worsen health habits.[80] It is often associated with avoidance of care and less exercise.[81] Furthermore, weight loss is strongly tied to later weight gain,[82] and weight cycling is a strong risk factor for increasing BMI and abdominal fat.[83] While these clinics think that they are helping, in fact they may be recommending the one thing *most* likely to cause additional long-term weight gain in women.

Given the high failure rate of many of the programs that promote postpartum weight loss in obese women,[84] a better approach may be the Health at Every Size paradigm. Research shows that it improves multiple health measures more sustainably than a traditional diet approach.[85]

Bariatric obstetrics is an appealing model in theory, but its reality is more ominous. It strips obese women of their right to patient autonomy, it funnels them into a high-cost and high-intervention care model, it subjects them to stigma and manipulative pressure to lose weight, and it may well end up making them heavier in the long run. Fat women deserve better.

Many well-meaning providers talk incessantly about the "teachable moment" that pregnancy provides.[86] They see it as a rare window of opportunity when a fat woman is willing to improve her habits for the sake of her unborn baby. They note the characteristics of effective teachable moments, including a "cueing event" that:[87]

1. Increases perceptions of personal risk and outcome expectancies
2. Prompts strong affective or emotional responses
3. Redefines self-concept or social role

In other words, scare the fat woman into believing that she and her baby are strongly at risk, take advantage of the emotional vulnerability around pregnancy, and play upon mother guilt by emphasizing her job to be a role model for her child.

A key part of this "teachable moment" is promoting the concept that "obesity begins in the womb." It's not enough to target fat kids or toddlers;[88] now they want to start targeting fetuses in utero.[89] As one article explains:[90]

> Scientists . . . worry about what are called epigenetic changes. The genes inherited from mother and father may be turned on and off and the strength of their effects changed by environmental conditions in early development. Many doctors are concerned about women being obese and unhealthy before pregnancy because, as they point out, the womb is the baby's first environment.

Doctors use the loaded image of babies "marinating" in an obesogenic, malevolent womb.[91] By using such manipulative language, doctors set the stage for justifying increasingly strong interventions in the pregnancies of obese women, including prenatal weight gain extremism.

The Institute of Medicine changed its guidelines in 2009 to suggest that obese women gain only 11 to 20 pounds and overweight women 15 to 25 pounds.[92] But many doctors don't think these guidelines go far enough. Dr. Raul Artal of the St. Louis Pregnancy Bariatric Clinic, for example, suggests that women gain no more than 10 pounds, and he pushes his "morbidly obese" patients to actually *lose* weight while pregnant.[93]

This is not an isolated trend. A look at headlines from media articles in the last few years shows that prenatal weight gain extremism is escalating:

- Doctors Urge Less Pregnancy Weight Gain for Obese Women[94]
- New Goal for the Obese: Zero Weight Gain in Pregnancy[95]
- Obese and Pregnant: Dieting Safe for Mom, Baby[96]
- It's Safe for Obese Moms-to-Be to Lose Weight during Pregnancy, New Research Finds[97]

While there is some research to support the idea that very large weight gains in obese women increase the risk for poor outcomes,[98] there is also research to support the idea that gaining very little weight or losing weight in pregnancy increases risks too.[99] For example, very low gain or gestational weight loss is associated with the risk for premature babies,[100] small-for-gestational-age babies (SGA babies),[101] neonatal intensive care unit admissions,[102] and stillbirth or infant death.[103]

Most obstetricians shrug off these risks, saying that the benefits far outbalance the risks. Yet SGA babies are at greater risk for many health issues later in life, including neurodevelopmental delay, insulin resistance, metabolic syndrome, and diabetes.[104] Disturbingly, SGA babies are also more at risk for stillbirth,[105] and some research shows that SGA babies of obese mothers are at particular risk.[106]

A recent Cochrane research review concluded, "Until the safety of weight loss in obese pregnant women can be established, there can be no practice recommendations for these women to intentionally lose weight during the pregnancy period."[107] Yet many women of size are being given extremist messages in the hopes that this will prevent pregnancy complications and future obesity:[108]

- I am pregnant with identical twin girls . . . [he told me] that I needed to lose 20 pounds during this pregnancy.
- If you don't lose 50 lbs. during pregnancy, you will have to have a cesarean and possibly a hysterectomy.
- My fat-phobic OB . . . put me on a 1000–1100 calorie a day diet with baby #4.
- You should eat nothing but vegetables for the rest of pregnancy.
- The OB told me, while pregnant with *twins*, to drink Slim-Fast . . . to keep down my weight gain.

Still other researchers are recruiting women into experimental trials to use medication to prevent so-called overweight Sumo babies.[109] Researchers in the UK are now experimenting with giving obese women the diabetes medication metformin during pregnancy in order to prevent big babies.[110] They theorize that many high-BMI women are insulin-resistant, so they hope that giving women metformin even when they are not diabetic may make their babies smaller and less prone to obesity later on.[111]

Although metformin has a good safety profile outside of pregnancy, its safety in pregnancy is less well known. It has been used successfully in diabetics and women with PCOS,[112] but these trials have been relatively small so far and many doctors urge caution with its use.[113]

We don't know the effect of using metformin in the pregnancies of women who don't need it. If this is intended to make babies smaller, what might be the effect in fat women who would have had average-sized fetuses anyhow? Will we be creating a whole new set of SGA babies with all their attendant health risks?

It is especially disturbing to see the widespread publicizing in the media of this metformin experiment in process. We won't know if this medication regimen was truly safe for many years, yet it is being promoted in the popular press as the next cure for obesity in the womb. This premarketing of an experiment still under way is premature and alarming.

The investigation of fetal programming in the womb is a fascinating field, but it is one that must be approached with great caution because of its lifelong implications. Experimenting on the fetuses of obese women is ethically questionable and is fraught with the possibility for abuse. Any work in this field must go slowly and carefully. It should *not* be used as the latest tool in fat eugenics.

The "anorexiation" of our babies must cease. Stop putting the baby on a diet before it's even born, and stop experimental extremism with fat pregnant women. Focus instead on excellent nutrition and emphasize regular, reasonable exercise. A healthy lifestyle may do much to address pregnancy issues with less danger to the baby and mother and fewer ethical quandaries.

The war on obesity regularly stigmatizes and blames fat people for their weight. As one author notes, "Society regularly regards obese persons not as innocent victims, but as architects of their own ill health, personally responsible for their weight problems because of laziness and overeating."[114] But this stigma reaches a whole new level of condemnation around the issue of obesity and pregnancy.

Recent public health messages are loaded with rhetoric about how dangerous pregnancy is at larger sizes and how much risk could be avoided if only fat women would stop being so irresponsible and just lose weight.[115] Barring that, fat women are supposed to be good patients by gaining next to nothing (or even losing) during pregnancy, submitting meekly to massive amounts of extra interventions for delivery, and taking experimental medication to eradicate obesity in the womb.

Many clinicians mean well when they employ draconian tactics like these with women of size; they want to help improve outcomes. The question is whether these care providers are doing more harm than good and whether their overbearing tactics are infringing on these women's rights to respectful care, patient autonomy, and indeed, their very right to procreate.

The troubling "blame-the-fat-mothers" meme in many of the messages around weight and pregnancy these days is tainted by underlying tinges of racism, classism, and sexism.[116] And they bring up important questions that society and ethicists need to spend more time contemplating.

For example, how far should society go to prevent obesity? Can it even be prevented in the first place? Should it? How much does the perceived burden on society justify the mistreatment of fat women during pregnancy? Does pressuring women to lose weight before pregnancy go far enough, or should they be guilted into having a gastric bypass first?[117] Should they be prosecuted for child abuse if they *don't* lose weight before pregnancy?[118] Should they be penalized by automatic cesarean if they gain too much weight in pregnancy?[119] Should fat women be prohibited altogether from having children?[120]

Deep down, many doctors want to keep fat women from procreating so they don't pass along their fat genes to the next generation. They want to be the gatekeepers of who is allowed to reproduce. If they can't do that, then they'll try to stop obesity in the womb by pressuring women to lose weight before pregnancy, to gain virtually nothing during pregnancy, or to take experimental medications during pregnancy.

The womb is now ground zero in the war on obesity.

This is fat eugenics, it is unjust and unethical, and it must stop.

NOTES

1. Joel Fuhrman, "Obesity during Pregnancy Puts the Child in Danger," *Disease Proof* (blog), April 6, 2010, accessed May 28, 2013, http://www.diseaseproof.com/archives/healthy-pregnancy-obesity-during-pregnancy-puts-the-child-in-danger.html; Annie Murphy Paul, "Too Fat and Pregnant," *New York Times Magazine*, July 13, 2008, accessed May 28, 2013, http://www.nytimes.com/2008/07/13/magazine/13wwln-essay-t.html?_r=0; "Get to a Healthy Weight Before Pregnancy," *cbsnews.com*, July 28, 2009, accessed June 2, 2013, http://www.cbsnews.com/2100-500398_162-5049469.html.

2. Lisa Collier Cool, "The #1 Pregnancy Risk," *Yahoo Health*, April 5, 2011, accessed May 29, 2013, http://health.yahoo.net/experts/dayinhealth/1-pregnancy-risk,.

3. Carey Goldberg, "10 Scary Reasons to Fight Obesity Before Pregnancy," *WBUR's Common Health Reform and Reality*, November 18, 2011, accessed May 27, 2013, http://commonhealth.wbur.org/2011/11/scary-reasons-obesity-pregnancy,.

4. Sue Dunlevy, "Fat Mothers Putting Babies' Health at Risk," *Courier Mail*, July 11, 2010, accessed May 31, 2013, http://www.couriermail.com.au/lifestyle/fat-mothers-putting-babies-health-at-risk/story-e6frer4f-1225890458554.

5. Maureen Cavanaugh and Pat Finn, "Pregnancy & Obesity: A Dangerous Combo," *KBPS* (podcast audio), June 20, 2010, accessed May 29, 2013, http://www.kpbs.org/news/2010/jun/30/pregnancy-obesity-dangerous-combo/.

6. V. A. Schmied et al. " 'Not Waving but Drowning': A Study of the Experiences and Concerns of Midwives and Other Health Professionals Caring for Obese Childbearing Women," *Midwifery* 27, no. 4 (August 2011): 424–30. doi: 10.1016/j.midw.2010.02.010, http://www.ncbi.nlm.nih.gov/pubmed/20381222; Claire Murphy, "Obesity in Pregnant Women Is a Ticking Time Bomb," *Herald.ie*, May 18, 2012, accessed May 29, 2013, http://www.herald.ie/lifestyle/health-beauty/obesity-in

-pregnant-women-is-a-ticking-timebomb-28008456.html; "Heavy Labor: Obesity and Pregnancy Are a Dangerous Mix," *Pittsburgh Post-Gazette*, June 17, 2010, accessed May 29, 2013, http://www.post-gazette.com/stories/opinion/editorials/heavy-labor -obesity-and-pregnancy-are-a-dangerous-mix-251663/.

7. Abe Sauer, "Real America, with Abe Sauer: Fat, Fetuses and Felonies," *The Awl*, October 14, 2009, accessed May 28, 2013, http://www.theawl.com/2009/10/real -america-with-abe-sauer-fat-fetuses-and-felonies.

8. Pamela Vireday, "Exaggerating the Risks Again," *The Well-Rounded Mama* (blog), June 10, 2010, accessed May 31, 2013, http://wellroundedmama.blogspot. com/2010/06/exaggerating-risks-again.html.

9. S. Joy et al., "The Impact of Maternal Obesity on the Incidence of Adverse Pregnancy Outcomes in High-Risk Term Pregnancies," *American Journal of Perinatology* 26, no. 5 (May 2009): 345–49, doi: 10.1055/s-0028-1110084, http:// www.ncbi.nlm.nih.gov/pubmed/19067282.

10. Pamela Vireday, "Rethinking the Obesity Paradigm: An Insider's View (Part One)," *Science and Sensibility* (blog), June 10, 2011, accessed May 28, 2013, http:// www.scienceandsensibility.org/?p=3030.

11. "Advice on Getting Pregnant—Obese Ladies Need to Lose Weight to Avoid Developmental Delays," www.whattoexpect.com (blog), March 12, 2012, accessed June 2, 2013, http://www.whattoexpect.com/blogs/librarianmommyreferencebookon parenting/advice-on-getting-pregnant-obese-ladies-need-to-lose-weight-to-avoid -developmental-delays; Sharon Kirkey, "Obesity in Pregnancy Putting Baby, Mom at Risk: Ottawa Study," *Vancouver Sun*, March 19, 2013, accessed May 28, 2013, http:// www.vancouversun.com/health/women/Obesity+pregnancy+putting+baby+risk +Ottawa+study/8119191/story.html.

12. Rachel Reilly, "Obese Mothers Who Have Weight-Loss Surgery Before Giving Birth Have Thinner Children, Say Researchers," *Mail Online*, May 28, 2013, accessed May 29, 2013, http://www.dailymail.co.uk/health/article-2332088/Should-obese -women-weight-loss-surgery-pregnancy-prevent-children-fat.html?ito=feeds-newsxml; Rebecca Smith, "Obese Pregnant Women Have More Complicated Births: Research," *Telegraph*, January 26, 2011, accessed May 29, 2013, http://www.telegraph.co.uk/ health/healthnews/8280720/Obese-pregnant-women-have-more-complicated-births -research.html; Kim I. Hartman, "Canada: Doctors Propose Denying Obese Women Fertility Treatments," *Digital Journal*, September 21, 2011, accessed May 27, 2013, http://digitaljournal.com/article/311789#ixzz1aLBiabvr.

13. C. A. Heuer, K. J. McClure, and R. M. Puhl, "Obesity Stigma in Online News: A Visual Content Analysis," *Journal of Health Communication* 16, no. 9 (October 2011): 976–87, doi: 10.1080/10810730.2011.561915, http://www.ncbi .nlm.nih.gov/pubmed/21541876; K. J. McClure, R. M. Puhl, and C. A. Heuer, "Obesity in the News: Do Photographic Images of Obese Persons Influence Antifat Attitudes?," *Journal of Health Communication* 16, no. 4 (April 2011): 359–71, doi: 10.1080/10810730.2010.535108, http://www.ncbi.nlm.nih.gov/pubmed/21181601; Arya M. Sharma, "People with Obesity Have Heads Too," *drsharma.ca* (blog), January 17, 2011, accessed June 2, 2013, http://www.drsharma.ca/people-with -obesity-have-heads-too.html.

14. Anemona Hartocollis, "Growing Obesity Increases the Perils of Childbearing," *New York Times*, June 5, 2010, accessed May 28, 2013, http://www.nytimes.com/2010/06/06/health/06obese.html?adxnnl=1&emc=eta1&adxnnlx=1307355101-XRbzrRQ+bFL/k/Go8IiKoA&_r=0.

15. Katie Moisse, "Obese and Pregnant: Dieting Safe for Mom, Baby," *abcnews.go.com*, May 18, 2012, accessed May 30, 2013, http://abcnews.go.com/Health/Wellness/obese-pregnant-dieting-safe-mom-baby/story?id=16371528#.UacV1JO1b5A.

16. Meredith Cohn, "Diets Suggested for More Pregnant Women," *Baltimore Sun*, June 24, 2012, accessed May 29, 2013, http://articles.baltimoresun.com/2012-06-24/health/bs-hs-obese-and-pregnant-20120624_1_pregnant-women-obesity-rates-normal-weight-women; Ann Dempsey, "Big Moms, Small Babes: Fitness Program Aims to Stop Childhood Obesity in Womb," *Fort Frances Times Online*, May 6, 2010, accessed May 30, 2013, http://www.fftimes.com/node/233322.

17. Dunlevy, "Fat Mothers Putting Babies' Health at Risk."

18. Ann M. Little, "Fat Is the New Crack," *Historiann* (blog), March 24, 2010, accessed May 28, 2013, http://www.historiann.com/2010/03/24/fat-is-the-new-crack/.

19. Paul Campos et al., "The Epidemiology of Overweight and Obesity: Public Health Crisis or Moral Panic?," *International Journal of Epidemiology* 35, no. 1 (2005): 55–60. doi: 10.1093/ije/dyi254, http://ije.oxfordjournals.org/content/35/1/55.

20. Elle, "Kindergartners, YOU'RE DOOMED!!!!" *Shakesville* (blog), March 23, 2010, accessed May 28, 2013, http://www.shakesville.com/2010/03/kindergarteners-youre-doomed.html; S. E. Gollust, I. Eboh, and C. L. Barry, "Picturing Obesity: Analyzing the Social Epidemiology of Obesity Conveyed through U.S. News Media Images," *Social Science & Medicine* 74, no. 10 (May 2012): 1544–51, doi: 10.1016/j.socscimed.2012.01.021, http://www.ncbi.nlm.nih.gov/pubmed/22445762.

21. Abigail C. Saguy and Kjerstin Gruys, "Morality and Health: News Media Constructions of Overweight and Eating Disorders," *Social Problems* 57, no. 2 (2010): 231–50, doi: 10.1525/sp.2010.57.2.231, http://www.sscnet.ucla.edu/soc/faculty/saguy/saguyandgruys.pdf.

22. Anemona Hartocollis, "Growing Obesity Increases the Perils of Childbearing," *New York Times*, June 5, 2010, accessed May 28, 2013, http://www.nytimes.com/2010/06/06/health/06obese.html?adxnnl=1&emc=eta1&adxnnlx=1307355101-XRbzrRQ+bFL/k/Go8IiKoA&_r=0; Meredith Cohn, "Diets Suggested for More Pregnant Women," *Baltimore Sun*, June 24, 2012, accessed May 29, 2013, http://articles.baltimoresun.com/2012-06-24/health/bs-hs-obese-and-pregnant-20120624_1_pregnant-women-obesity-rates-normal-weight-women.

23. Jeanne Firth, "Healthy Choices and Heavy Burdens: Race, Citizenship and Gender in the 'Obesity Epidemic,'" *Journal of International Women's Studies* 13, no. 2 (March 2012): 33–50, accessed May 30, 2013, http://www.bridgew.edu/soas/jiws/Vol13_no2/Article3.pdf.

24. Pamela Vireday, "Care Providers vs. 'Scare' Providers," *The Well-Rounded Mama* (blog), May 13, 2009, accessed May 28, 2013, http://wellroundedmama.blogspot.com/2009/05/care-providers-vs-scare-providers.html.

25. Dunlevy, "Fat Mothers Putting Babies' Health at Risk."

26. E. Jarvie and J. E. Ramsay, "Obstetric Management of Obesity in Pregnancy," *Seminars in Fetal and Neonatal Medicine* 15, no. 2 (April 2010): 83–88, doi: 10.1016/j.siny.2009.10.001, http://www.ncbi.nlm.nih.gov/pubmed/19880362.

27. Pamela Vireday, "Rethinking the Obesity Paradigm: An Insider's View (Part One)," *Science and Sensibility* (blog), June 10, 2011, accessed May 28, 2013, http://www.scienceandsensibility.org/?p=3030.

28. Pamela Vireday, "Exaggerating the Risks Again," *The Well-Rounded Mama* (blog), June 10, 2010, accessed May 31, 2013, http://wellroundedmama.blogspot.com/2010/06/exaggerating-risks-again.html.

29. "Fat Pregnancy Equals Death?," *The Well-Rounded Mama* (blog), June 8, 2008, accessed May 28, 2013, http://www.wellroundedmama.blogspot.com/2008/06/fat-pregnancy-equals-death.html; "If You Get Pregnant You Will Gestational Diabetes, Have High Blood Pressure . . . and . . . Die," *My OB Said WHAT?!?* (blog), March 12, 2010, accessed May 29, 2013, http://myobsaidwhat.com/2010/03/12/if-you-get-pregnant-you-will-get-gestational-diabetes-have-high-blood-pressure-and-die/; Vireday, "Care Providers vs. 'Scare' Providers."

30. Vireday, "Care Providers vs. 'Scare' Providers"; "Fat Pregnancy Equals Death?"

31. "Pressure for Abortion for Obese Women," *The Well-Rounded Mama* (blog), June 15, 2008, accessed May 28, 2013, http://wellroundedmama.blogspot.com/2008/06/pressure-for-abortion-for-obese-women.html; Pamela Vireday, "Please Document Your Stories of Mistreatment," *The Well-Rounded Mama* (blog), August 23, 2010, accessed May 27, 2013, http://wellroundedmama.blogspot.com/2010/08/please-document-your-stories-of.html; "Too Old and Too Fat to Be Pregnant (FFS!)," *First, Do No Harm* (blog), n.d., accessed May 31, 2013, http://fathealth.wordpress.com/2013/02/03/too-old-and-too-fat-to-be-pregnant-ffs/.

32. "Gina Marie's Story," *The Well-Rounded Mama* (blog), June 2008, accessed May 28, 2013, http://www.wellroundedmama.blogspot.com/2008/06/gina-maries-story.html.

33. "Adoption and People of Size," *The Well-Rounded Mama* (blog), January 19, 2009, accessed May 28, 2013, http://www.wellroundedmama.blogspot.com/2009/01/adoption-and-people-of-size.html.

34. "ACOG Committee Opinion: Obesity in Pregnancy," *The American Congress of Obstetricians and Gynecologists*, no. 549 (January 2013), accessed May 29, 2013, http://www.acog.org/Resources%20And%20Publications/Committee%20Opinions/Committee%20on%20Obstetric%20Practice/Obesity%20in%20Pregnancy.aspx.

35. Rebecca Smith, "Obese Women 'Should Lose Weight' Before Having a Baby," *Telegraph*, December 22, 2011, accessed May 29, 2013, http://www.telegraph.co.uk/health/healthnews/8969907/Obese-women-should-lose-weight-before-having-a-baby.html; Scott Hensley, "Obese English Women Told to Cut Calories Before Pregnancy," *npr.org* (blog), July 28, 2010, accessed May 29, 2013, http://www.npr.org/blogs/health/2010/07/28/128817182/obese-english-women-told-to-cut-calories-before-pregnancy.

36. Rebecca Smith, "Obese Pregnant Women 'Putting Health at Risk,'" *Telegraph*, December 7, 2010, accessed May 29, 2013, http://www.telegraph.co.uk/health/healthnews/8184045/Obese-pregnant-women-putting-health-at-risk.html; "Study:

Lose Weight Before Pregnancy," *Medical Daily*, April 13, 2012, accessed May 29, 2013, http://www.medicaldaily.com/articles/9519/20120413/obesity-maternal -obesity-pregnancy-research.htm.

37. D. Getahun et al., "Changes in Prepregnancy Body Mass Index between the First and Second Pregnancies and Risk of Large-for-Gestational-Age Birth," *Obstetrics and Gynecology* 196, no. 6 (December 2007): 530.e1–8, http://www.ncbi .nlm.nih.gov/pubmed/17547882; V. E. Whiteman et al., "Changes in Prepregnancy Body Mass Index between Pregnancies and Risk of Gestational and Type 2 Diabetes," *Archives of Gynecology and Obstetrics* 284, no. 1 (July 2011): 235–40, doi: 10.1007/s00404-011-1917-7, http://www.ncbi.nlm.nih.gov/pubmed/21544736; D. Mostello et al., "Recurrent Preeclampsia: The Effect of Weight Change between Pregnancies," *Obstetrics and Gynecology* 116, no. 3 (September 2010): 667–72, doi: 10.1097/AOG.0b013e3181ed74ea, http://www.ncbi.nlm.nih.gov/pubmed/20733450.

38. L. Suarez et al., "Dieting to Lose Weight and Occurrence of Neural Tube Defects in Offspring of Mexican-American Women," *Maternal and Child Health Journal* 15, no. 4 (May 2012): 844–49, doi: 10.1007/s10995-011-0806-9, http://www .ncbi.nlm.nih.gov/pubmed/21512779; S. L. Carmichael et al., "Dieting Behaviors and Risk of Neural Tube Defects," *American Journal of Epidemiology* 158, no. 12 (December 15, 2003): 1127–31, http://www.ncbi.nlm.nih.gov/pubmed/14652296.

39. P. Paramsothy et al., "Interpregnancy Weight Gain and Cesarean Delivery Risk in Women with a History of Gestational Diabetes," *Obstetrics and Gynecology* 113, no. 4 (April 2009): 817–23. doi: 10.1097/AOG.0b013e31819b33ac, http://www .ncbi.nlm.nih.gov/pubmed/19305325; N. L. Glazer et al., "Weight Change and the Risk of Gestational Diabetes in Obese Women," *Epidemiology* 15, no. 6 (November 2004): 733–37, http://www.ncbi.nlm.nih.gov/pubmed/15475723; S. L. Mumford et al., "Dietary Restraint and Gestational Weight Gain," *Journal of the American Dietary Association* 108, no. 10 (October 2008): 1646–53, doi: 10.1016/ j.jada.2008.07.016, http://www.ncbi.nlm.nih.gov/pubmed/18926129.

40. N. J. Jain et al., "Maternal Obesity: Can Pregnancy Weight Gain Modify Risk of Selected Adverse Pregnancy Outcomes?," *American Journal of Perinatology* 24, no. 5 (May 2007): 291–98, http://www.ncbi.nlm.nih.gov/pubmed/17514601.

41. "Methods for Voluntary Weight Loss and Control," NIH Technology Assessment Conference Panel, *Annals of Internal Medicine* 116, no. 11 (June 1992): 942–99, http://www.ncbi.nlm.nih.gov/pubmed/1580453.

42. W. C. Miller, "How Effective Are Traditional Dietary and Exercise Interventions for Weight Loss?," *Medicine and Science in Sports and Exercise* 31, no. 8 (August 1999): 1129–34, http://www.ncbi.nlm.nih.gov/pubmed/10449014; D. Crawford, R. W. Jeffery, and S. A. French, "Can Anyone Successfully Control Their Weight? Findings of a Three Year Community-Based Study of Men and Women,"*International Journal of Obesity and Related Metabolic Disorders* 24, no. 9 (September 2000): 1107–10, http://www.ncbi.nlm.nih.gov/ pubmed/11033978.

43. T. Mann et al., "Medicare's Search for Effective Obesity Treatments: Diets Are Not the Answer," *The American Psychologist* 62, no. 3 (April 2007): 220–33, http:// www.ncbi.nlm.nih.gov/pubmed/17469900/.

44. J. D. Douketis et al., "Systematic Review of Long-Term Weight Loss Studies in Obese Adults: Clinical Significance and Applicability to Clinical Practice," *International Journal of Obesity (London)* 29, no. 10 (October 2005): 1153–67, http://www.ncbi.nlm.nih.gov/pubmed/15997250.

45. J. Guest et al., "Evidence for Under-Nutrition in Adolescent Females Using Routine Dieting Practices," *Asia Pacific Journal of Clinical Nutrition* 19, no. 4 (2010): 526–33, http://www.ncbi.nlm.nih.gov/pubmed/21147714; M. J. Kretsch et al., "Cognitive Function, Iron Status, and Hemoglobin Concentration in Obese Dieting Women," *European Journal of Clinical Nutrition* 52, no. 7 (July 1998): 512–18, http://www.ncbi.nlm.nih.gov/pubmed/9683334.

46. Polly Curtis, "Infertility Crisis Looms in the West as Obesity Levels Soar," *Guardian*, August 23, 2007, accessed May 27, 2013, http://www.guardian.co.uk/society/2007/aug/24/health.healthandwellbeing; Zulehkha Waheed, "Ban on Fertility Treatment for Obese Women Proposed," *IVF.net*, April 11, 2007, accessed May 27, 2013, http://www.ivf.net/ivf/ban-on-fertility-treatment-for-obese-women-proposed-o2632.html.

47. Vireday, "Please Document Your Stories of Mistreatment"; "Fat Women Only Have Babies Because We Can't Stop Them," *My OB Said WHAT?!?* (blog), April 19, 2013, accessed May 27, 2013, http://myobsaidwhat.com/2013/04/19/fat-women-only-have-babies-because-we-cant-stop-them/; Shawna Cohen, "Are You Too Fat for Fertility Treatments?," *Mommyish.com*, September 22, 2011, accessed May 31, 2013, http://www.mommyish.com/2011/09/22/are-you-too-fat-for-fertility-treatments-338/.

48. Anjel Vahratian and Yolanda R. Smith, "Should Access to Fertility-Related Services Be Conditional on Body Mass Index?," *Human Reproduction* 24, no. 7 (July 2009): 1532–37, doi: 10.1093/humrep/dep057, http://www.ncbi.nlm.nih.gov/pmc/articles/PMC2698326/.

49. A. Maheshwari et al., "Direct Health Services Costs of Providing Assisted Reproduction Services in Older Women," *Fertility and Sterility* 93, no. 2 (February 2010): 527–36, doi: 10.1016/j.fertnstert.2009.01.115, http://www.ncbi.nlm.nih.gov/pubmed/19261279.

50. "You're Hugely Fat," *My OB Said WHAT?!?* (blog), April 17, 2013, accessed May 27, 2013, http://myobsaidwhat.com/2013/04/17/youre-hugely-fat/.

51. Kim I. Hartman, "Canada: Doctors Propose Denying Obese Women Fertility Treatments," *Digital Journal*, September 21, 2011, accessed May 27, 2013, http://digitaljournal.com/article/311789#ixzz1aLBiabvr.

52. Brooke LeMaster, "Medical Advice about Becoming Pregnant," *tudiabetes.org*, July 15, 2009, accessed May 31, 2013, http://www.tudiabetes.org/group/ohbaby/forum/topics/medical-advice-about-becoming?page=1&commentId=583967%3AComment%3A751024&x=1; Stephen A. Paget, "Use of Fertility Drugs in Patients with Systemic Autoimmunity," *Medscape Today News*, June 26, 2003, accessed May 31, 2013, http://www.medscape.com/viewarticle/457058; "Fertility Treatment Hormones with Clotting Disorders?," *community.babycenter.com*, April 27, 2011, accessed May 31, 2013, http://community.babycenter.com/post/a27446091/fertility_treatment_hormomes_w_clotting_disorders.

53. A. H. Goris and K. R. Westerterp, "Physical Activity, Fat Intake and Body Fat," *Physiology & Behavior*, 94, no. 2 (May 23, 2008): 164–68, http://www.ncbi.nlm.nih.gov/pubmed/18068203.

54. Anemona Hartocollis, "Growing Obesity Increases the Perils of Childbearing," *New York Times*, June 5, 2010, accessed May 28, 2013, http://www.nytimes.com/2010/06/06/health/06obese.html?adxnnl=1&emc=eta1&adxnnlx=1307355101-XRbzrRQ+bFL/k/Go8IiKoA&_r=0.

55. Pamela Vireday, "Reply Turned Post: Ghettoizing Fat Pregnant Women," *The Well-Rounded Mama* (blog), December 2, 2009, accessed May 31, 2013, http://wellroundedmama.blogspot.com/2009/12/reply-turned-post-ghettoizing-fat.html.

56. Bob LaMendola, "Some Ob-Gyns in South Florida Turn Away Overweight Women," *Sun Sentinel*, May 16, 2011, accessed May 30, 2013, http://articles.sun-sentinel.com/2011-05-16/health/fl-hk-no-obesity-doc-20110516_1_gyn-ob-gyn-obese-patients.

57. Richard Savill, "Fat Mothers to Be Banned from Hospital," *Telegraph*, November 12, 2009, accessed May 31, 2013, http://www.telegraph.co.uk/health/healthnews/6555422/Fat-mothers-to-be-banned-from-hospital.html; "South Australian Perinatal Practice Guidelines: Women with a High Body Mass Index," *South Australian Perinatal Practice Guidelines Workgroup*, 978-1-74243-273-1, last updated November 20, 2012, http://www.health.sa.gov.au/PPG/Default.aspx?PageContentMode=1&tabid=77.

58. Lynne Jeter, "Stemming the Obesity Epidemic: SLU Department Chair Develops Missouri's First Special Obstetrics Program," *St. Louis Medical News*, accessed May 29, 2013, http://saintlouismedicalnews.com/content/stemming-obesity-epidemic; Jeannine M. Cobb, "Obesity and Pregnancy: The Bariatrician's Role," *MD News*, June 29, 2011, accessed May 29, 2013, http://www.mdnews.com/news/2011_06/05849_may2011_obesity-and-pregnancy.aspx.

59. Jacqueline Stenson, "Eating for Two, Gaining Too Much," *Los Angeles Times*, August 22, 2005, accessed June 5, 2013, http://articles.latimes.com/2005/aug/22/health/he-pregnancy22.

60. K. Mulherin et al., "Weight Stigma in Maternity Care: Women's Experiences and Care Providers' Attitudes," *BMC Pregnancy and Childbirth* 13 (January 22, 2013): 19, doi: 10.1186/1471-2393-13-19, http://www.biomedcentral.com/content/pdf/1471-2393-13-19.pdf.

61. Vireday, "Reply Turned Post."

62. J. L. Weiss et al., "Obesity, Obstetric Complications and Cesarean Delivery Rate—a Population-Based Screening Study," *American Journal of Obstetrics and Gynecology* 190, no. 4 (April 2004): 1091–97, http://www.ncbi.nlm.nih.gov/pubmed/15118648; B. C. Brost et al., "The Preterm Prediction Study: Association of Cesarean Delivery with Increases in Maternal Weight and Body Mass Index," *American Journal of Obstetrics and Gynecology* 177, no. 2 (August 1997): 333–37, http://www.ncbi.nlm.nih.gov/pubmed/9290448; B. P. Wispelwey and E. Sheiner, "Cesarean Delivery in Obese Women: A Comprehensive Review," *Journal of Maternal, Fetal and Neonatal Medicine* 26, no. 6 (April 2013): 547–51, doi: 10.3109/14767058.2012.745506, http://www.ncbi.nlm.nih.gov/pubmed/23130683.

63. Pamela Vireday, "Please Document Your Stories of Mistreatment," *The Well-Rounded Mama Blog*. http://wellroundedmama.blogspot.com/2010/08/please -document-your-stories-of.html, Monday August 23, 2010. Accessed on 5/27/13 at 8:15 p.m.

64. R. M. Silver et al., "Maternal Morbidity Associated with Multiple Repeat Cesarean Deliveries," *Obstetrics and Gynecology* 107, no. 6 (June 2006): 1226–32, http://www.ncbi.nlm.nih.gov/pubmed/16738145.

65. "New Study Reveals Midwife-Led Birth Centers a Key to Decreased Cesarean Rate, Lower Health Costs," *birthwithoutfearblog.com* (blog), January 31, 2013, accessed June 2, 2013, http://birthwithoutfearblog.com/2013/01/31/new-study-reveals-midwife -led-birth-centers-a-key-to-decreased-cesarean-rate-lower-health-care-costs/; P. A. Janssen et al., "Outcomes of Planned Hospital Birth Attended by Midwives Compared with Physicians in British Columbia,"*Birth* 34, no. 2 (June 2007): 140–47, http://www.ncbi.nlm.nih.gov/pubmed/17542818; T. L. King, "Preventing Primary Cesarean Sections: Intrapartum Care," *Seminars in Perinatology* 36, no. 5 (October 2012): 357–64, doi: 10.1053/j.semperi.2012.04.020, http://www.ncbi.nlm .nih.gov/pubmed/23009969.

66. L. Cragin and H. P. Kennedy, "Linking Obstetric and Midwifery Practice with Optimal Outcomes," *Journal of Obstetric, Gynecological and Neonatal Nursing* 35, no. 6 (November–December 2006): 779–85, http://www.ncbi.nlm.nih.gov/pubmed/ 17105644.

67. "Right to Midwife Led Unit for Women with High BMI," *babyand bump.momtastic.com*, December 20, 2011, accessed May 31, 2013, http:// babyandbump.momtastic.com/pregnancy-third-trimester/831227-right-midwife-led -unit-women-high-bmi.html; "Because of Your Weight ... We're Going to ... Schedule Your Cesarean," *My OB Said What?!?* (blog), June 21, 2011, accessed May 27, 2013, http://myobsaidwhat.com/2011/06/21/because-of-your -weigt-were-going-to-schedule-your-cesarean/; "Pregnancy and Doctor Doom— He Was Wrong, Wrong, Wrong!," *First, Do No Harm* (blog), May 10, 2010, accessed June 2, 2013, http://fathealth.wordpress.com/2010/05/10/pregnancy-and -doctor-doom-he-was-wrong-wrong-wrong/.

68. C. S. Homer et al., "Planned Vaginal Delivery or Planned Caesarean Delivery in Women with Extreme Obesity," *BJOG: An international Journal of Obstetrics and Gynaecology* 118, no. 4 (March 2011): 480–87, doi: 10.1111/j.1471-0528.2010 .02832.x, http://www.ncbi.nlm.nih.gov/pubmed/21244616; Vireday, "Please Document Your Stories of Mistreatment"; Comment from *My OB Said What?!?* (blog), June 21, 2011, accessed May 27, 2013, http://myobsaidwhat.com/2011/06/21/ because-of-your-weigt-were-going-to-schedule-your-cesarean/.

69. Homer et al., "Planned Vaginal Delivery or Planned Cesarean Delivery."

70. Pamela Vireday, "Routine Cesarean Not Better for 'Extreme Obesity,'" *The Well-Rounded Mama* (blog), April 18, 2011, accessed June 5, 2013, http:// wellroundedmama.blogspot.com/2011/04/routine-cesareans-not-better-for.html,.

71. H. A. Abenhaim et al., "Higher Cesarean Rates in Women with Higher Body Mass Index: Are We Managing Labour Differently?," *Journal of Obstetrics and Gynaecology Canada* 33, no. 5 (May 2011): 443–48, http://www.ncbi.nlm.nih.gov/

21639963; Pamela Vireday, "Healthy Birth Practices: Avoid Unnecessary Interventions," *The Well-Rounded Mama* (blog), January 31, 2010, accessed June 7, 2013, http://wellroundedmama.blogspot.com/2010/01/healthy-birth-practices-avoid .html.

72. T. S. Usha Kiran et al., "Outcome of Pregnancy in a Woman with an Increased Body Mass Index," *BJOG: An International Journal of Obstetrics and Gynaecology* 112, no. 6 (June 2005): 768–72, http://www.ncbi.nlm.nih.gov/pubmed/15924535.

73. C. Green and D. Shaker, "Impact of Morbid Obesity on the Mode of Delivery and Obstetric Outcome in Nulliparous Singleton Pregnancy and the Implications for Rural Maternity Services," *Australia and New Zealand Journal of Obstetrics and Gynaecology* 51, no. 2 (April 2011): 172–74, doi: 10.1111/j.1479-828X.2010 .01271.x, http://www.ncbi.nlm.nih.gov/pubmed/21466521; M. J. Garabedian et al., "Extreme Morbid Obesity and Labor Outcome in Nulliparous Women at Term," *American Journal of Perinataology* 28, no. 9 (October 2011): 729–34, doi: 10.1055/ s-0031-1280852, http://www.ncbi.nlm.nih.gov/pubmed/21660900.

74. "Problems and Hazards of Induction of Labor: A CIMS Fact Sheet," *dona.org*, accessed June 2, 2013, http://www.dona.org/PDF/CIMSinduct-fact-sheet.pdf.

75. Green and Shaker, "Impact of Morbid Obesity."

76. N. Farah et al., "Maternal Morbid Obesity and Obstetric Outcomes," *Obesity Facts 2*, no. 6 (2009): 352–54, doi: 10.1159/000261951, http://www.ncbi.nlm.nih. gov/pubmed/20090385.

77. Pamela Vireday, "Supersized Women and Cesareans: A Tale of Two Cities," *The Well-Rounded Mama* (blog), May 1, 2012, accessed June 4, 2013, http://well roundedmama.blogspot.com/2012/01/supersized-women-and-cesareans-tale-of.html.

78. Sarah Davies and Lynne Swann, "The Role of the Midwife in Improving Normal Birth Rates in Obese Women," *British Journal of Midwifery* 20, no. 1 (January 2012): 7–12, http://www.intermid.co.uk/cgi-bin/go.pl/library/abstract.html? uid=88769; Cathy Warwick, "Cathy Warwick Comments on the Overestimation of Risk during Pregnancy Relating to Weight Management, Obesity, and Normal Birth," *The Royal College of Midwives*, Press Release on October 17, 2010, accessed June 7, 2013, http://tinyurl.com/cms5q.

79. "Fat Pregnancy Equals Death?"; "Gina Marie's Story."

80. R. M. Puhl, C. A. Moss-Racusin, and M. B. Schwartz, "Internalization of Weight Bias: Implications for Binge-Eating and Emotional Well-Being," *Obesity (Silver Spring, Md.)* 15, no. 1 (January 2007): 19–23, http://www.ncbi.nlm.nih.gov/ pubmed/17228027/; L. R. Vartanian and J. M. Smyth, "Primum Non Nocere: Obesity Stigma and Public Health," *Journal of Bioethics Inquiry* 10, no. 1 (March 2013): 49–57, doi: 10.1007/s11673-012-9412-9, http://www.ncbi.nlm.nih .gov/pubmed/23288439; R. M. Puhl and C. A. Heuer, "Obesity Stigma: Important Considerations for Public Health," *American Journal of Public Health* 100, no. 6 (June 2010): 1019–28, doi: 10.2105/AJPH.2009, http://www.ncbi.nlm.nih.gov/ pubmed/20075322.

81. L. R. Vartanian and J. G. Shaprow, "Effects of Weight Stigma on Exercise Motivation and Behavior: A Preliminary Investigation among College-Aged Females," *Journal of Health Psychology* 13, no. 1 (January 2008): 131–38, http://www

.ncbi.nlm.nih.gov/pubmed/18086724/; L. R. Vartanian and S. A. Novak, "Internalized Societal Attitudes Moderate the Impact of Weight Stigma on Avoidance of Exercise," *Obesity (Silver Spring, Md.)* 19, no. 4 (April 2011): 757–62, doi: 10.1038/oby.2010.234, http://www.ncbi.nlm.nih.gov/pubmed/20948515; C. A. Drury and M. Louis, "Exploring the Association between Body Weight, Stigma of Obesity, and Health Care Avoidance," *Journal of the American Academy of Nurse Practitioners* 14, no. 12 (December 2002): 554–61, http://www.ncbi.nlm.nih.gov/pubmed/12567923.

82. Mann et al., "Medicare's Search for Effective Obesity Treatments"; P. D. Martin et al., "Weight Loss Maintenance Following a Primary Care Intervention for Low-Income Minority Women," *Obesity (Silver Spring, Md.)* 15, no. 11 (November 2008): 2462–67, doi: 10.1038/oby.2008.399, http://www.ncbi.nlm.nih.gov/pubmed/18787526.

83. A. E. Field et al., "Weight Cycling and the Risk of Developing Type 2 Diabetes among Adult Women in the United States," *Obesity Research* 12, no. 2 (February 2004): 267–74, http://www.ncbi.nlm.nih.gov/pubmed/14981219; E. Cereda et al., "Weight Cycling Is Associated with Body Weight Excess and Abdominal Fat Accumulation: A Cross-Sectional Study," *Clinical Nutrition* 30, no. 6 (December 2011): 718–23, doi: 10.1016/j.clnu.2011.06.009, http://www.ncbi.nlm.nih.gov/pubmed/21764186.

84. G. A. Wiltheiss et al., "Diet Quality and Weight Change among Overweight and Obese Postpartum Women Enrolled in a Behavioral Intervention Program," *Journal of the Academy of Nutrition and Dietetics* 113, no. 1 (January 2013): 54–62, doi: 10.1016/j.jand.2012.08.012, http://www.ncbi.nlm.nih.gov/pubmed/23146549; T. Østbye et al., "Active Mothers Postpartum: A Randomized Controlled Weight-Loss Intervention Trial," *American Journal of Preventive Medicine* 37, no. 3 (September 2009): 17380, doi: 10.1016/j.amepre.2009.05.016, http://www.ncbi.nlm.nih.gov/pubmed/19595557.

85. L. Bacon et al., "Size Acceptance and Intuitive Eating Improve Health for Obese, Female Chronic Dieters," *Journal of the American Dietetic Association* 105, no. 6 (June 2005): 929–36, http://www.ncbi.nlm.nih.gov/pubmed/15942543.

86. Suzanne Phelan, "Pregnancy: A 'Teachable Moment' for Weight Control and Obesity Prevention," *American Journal of Obstetrics and Gynecology* 202, no. 2 (February 2010): 135.e1–8, doi: 10.1016/j.ajog.2009.06.008, accessed May 29, 2013, http://digitalcommons.calpoly.edu/cgi/viewcontent.cgi?article=1043&context=kine_fac.

87. C. M. McBride, K. M. Emmons, and I. M. Lipkus, "Understanding the Potential of Teachable Moments: The Case of Smoking Cessation," *Health Education Research*, 18, no. 2 (April 2003): 156–70, accessed May 29, 2013, http://www.ncbi.nlm.nih.gov/pubmed/12729175.

88. Daniel Engber, "Leave the Fat Kids Alone: Efforts to Fix Childhood Obesity Are Aiming at the Wrong Target," *hive.slate.com*, March 10, 2011, accessed May 31, 2013, http://hive.slate.com/hive/time-to-trim/article/leave-the-fat-kids-alone; Margaret (Peggy) Bentley, "Mothers and Others: Family-Based Obesity Prevention for Infants and Toddlers," *UNC School of Medicine: Center for Women's Health Research at UNC*, accessed May 30, 2013, https://www.med.unc.edu/cwhr/research/

research-studies-ongoing-2/research-grants/mothers-and-others-family-based-obesity
-prevention-for-infants-and-toddlers.

89. P. D. Taylor and L. Poston, "Developmental Programming of Obesity in Mammals," *Experimental Physiology* 92, no. 2 (March 2007): 287–98, http://www
.ncbi.nlm.nih.gov/pubmed/17170060.

90. Roni Caryn Rabin, "Baby Fat May Not Be So Cute After All," *New York Times*, March 22, 2010, accessed May 28, 2013, http://www.nytimes.com/2010/03/23/health/
23obese.html?src=me&ref=general&_r=0.

91. Little, "Fat Is the New Crack"; Reilly, "Obese Mothers Who Have Weight-Loss Surgery"; "Obese Women Lose Weight Before Pregnancy," *UPI.com*, April 13, 2012, accessed May 29, 2013, http://www.upi.com/Health_News/2012/04/13/Obese
-women-lose-weight-before-pregnancy/UPI-34581334371213/.

92. Kathleen Kingsbury, "Tough Weight Guidelines for Obese Mothers-to-Be," *Time.com*, May 28, 2009, accessed May 29, 2013, http://www.time.com/time/health/
article/0,8599,1901441,00.html.

93. Michele Munz, "Obesity and Pregnancy Guidelines Stir Debate," *St. Louis Post-Dispatch*, July 6, 2011, accessed May 29, 2013, http://www.stltoday.com/lifestyles/
health-med-fit/fitness/obesity-and-pregnancy-guidelines-stir-debate/article_c4364887
-d53a-5bc7-8ccc-2485e43344dc.html.

94. Lauren Neergaard, "Doctors Urge Less Pregnancy Weight Gain for Obese Women," *boston.com*, May 29, 2009, accessed May 30, 2013, http://www.boston
.com/news/health/articles/2009/05/29/doctors_urge_less_pregnancy_weight_gain_for
_obese_women/.

95. Roni Caryn Rabin, "New Goal for the Obese: Zero Gain in Pregnancy," *New York Times*, December 14, 2009, accessed May 30, 2013, http://www.nytimes.com/
2009/12/15/health/15obese.html.

96. Katie Moisse, "Obese and Pregnant: Dieting Safe for Mom, Baby," *abcnews.go.com*, May 18, 2012, accessed May 30, 2013, http://abcnews.go.com/
Health/Wellness/obese-pregnant-dieting-safe-mom-baby/story?id=16371528#.UacV1
JO1b5A.

97. "It's Safe for Obese Moms-to-Be to Lose Weight during Pregnancy, New Research Finds," *Science Daily.com*, June 6, 2007, accessed May 30, 2013, http://www
.sciencedaily.com/releases/2007/06/070605185550.htm.

98. J. M. Crane et al., "The Effect of Gestational Weight Gain by Body Mass Index on Maternal and Neonatal Outcomes," *Journal of Obstetricians and Gynaecologists Canada* 31, no. 1 (January 2009): 28–35, http://www.ncbi.nlm.nih.gov/pubmed/
19208280; D. W. Kiel et al., "Gestational Weight Gain and Pregnancy Outcomes in Obese Women: How Much Is Enough?," *Obstetrics and Gynecology* 110, no. 4 (October 2007): 752–58, http://www.ncbi.nlm.nih.gov/pubmed/17906005.

99. A. Beyerlein et al., "Associations of Gestational Weight Loss with Birth-Related Outcome: A Retrospective Cohort Study," *BJOG: An International Journal of Obstetrics and Gynaecology* 118, no. 1 (January 2011): 55–61, doi: 10.1111/j.1471-0528
.2010.02761.x, http://www.ncbi.nlm.nih.gov/pubmed/21054761; L. E. Edwards et al.,
"Pregnancy Complications and Birth Outcomes in Obese and Normal-Weight Women: Effects of Gestational Weight Change," *Obstetrics and Gynecology* 87, no. 3

(March 1996): 389–94, http://www.ncbi.nlm.nih.gov/pubmed/8598961; L. M. Bodnar et al., "Severe Obesity, Gestational Weight Gain, and Adverse Birth Outcomes," *The American Journal of Clinical Nutrition* 91, no. 6 (June 2010): 1642–48, doi: 10.3945/ajcn.2009.29008, http://www.ncbi.nlm.nih.gov/pubmed/20357043.

100. P. M. Dietz et al., "Combined Effects of Prepregnancy Body Mass Index and Weight Gain During Pregnancy on the Risk of Preterm Delivery," *Epidemiology* 17, no. 2 (March 2006): 170–77, http://www.ncbi.nlm.nih.gov/pubmed/16477257; E. A. Nohr et al., "Obesity, Gestational Weight Gain and Preterm Birth: A Study within the Danish National Birth Cohort," *Paediatric and Perinatal Epidemiology* 21, no. 1 (January 2007): 5–14, http://www.ncbi.nlm.nih.gov/pubmed/17239174.

101. Bodnar et al., "Severe Obesity, Gestational Weight Gain, and Adverse Birth Outcomes"; K. K. Vesco et al., "Newborn Size among Obese Women with Weight Gain Outside the 2009 Institute of Medicine Recommendation," *Obstetrics and Gynecology* 117, no. 4 (April 2011): 812–18, doi: 10.1097/AOG.0b013e3182113ae4, http://www.ncbi.nlm.nih.gov/pubmed/21422851.

102. S. Potti et al., "Obstetric Outcomes in Normal Weight and Obese Women in Relation to Gestational Weight Gain: Comparison between Institute of Medicine Guidelines and Cedergren Criteria," *American Journal of Perinatology* 27, no. 5 (May 2010): 415–420, doi: 10.1055/s-0029-1243369, http://www.ncbi.nlm.nih.gov/pubmed/20013574.

103. A. Chen et al., "Maternal Obesity and the Risk of Infant Death in the United States," *Epidemiology* 20, no. 1 (January 2009): 74–81, doi: 10.1097/EDE.0b013e3181878645, http://www.ncbi.nlm.nih.gov/pubmed/18813025; R. L. Naeye, "Weight Gain and the Outcome of Pregnancy," *American Journal of Obstetrics and Gynecology* 135, no. 1 (September 1, 1979): 3–9, http://www.ncbi.nlm.nih.gov/pubmed/474659.

104. T. Arcangeli et al., "Neurodevelopmental Delay in Small Babies at Term: A Systematic Review," *Ultrasound in Obstetrics & Gynecology: The Official Journal of the International Society of Ultrasound in Obstetrics and Gynecology* 40, no. 3 (September 2012): 267–75, doi: 10.1002/uog.11112, http://www.ncbi.nlm.nih.gov/pubmed/22302630; T. Meas et al., "Independent Effects of Weight Gain and Fetal Programming on Metabolic Complications in Adults Born Small for Gestational Age," *Diabetologia* 53, no. 5 (May 2010): 907–13, doi: 10.1007/s00125-009-1650-y, http://www.ncbi.nlm.nih.gov/pubmed/20111856; A. Vaag et al., "Metabolic Aspects of Insulin Resistance in Individuals Born Small for Gestational Age," *Hormone Research* 65, Supplement 3 (2006): 137–43, http://www.ncbi.nlm.nih.gov/pubmed/16612127.

105. S. Vashevnik, S. Walker, and M. Permezel, "Stillbirths and Neonatal Deaths in Appropriate, Small and Large Birthweight for Gestational Age Fetuses," *Australia and New Zealand Journal of Obstetrics and Gynaecology* 47, no. 4 (August 2007): 302–6, http://www.ncbi.nlm.nih.gov/pubmed/17627685.

106. H. M. Salihu et al., "Success of Programming Fetal Growth Phenotypes among Obese Women," *Obstetrics and Gynecology* 114, no. 2, pt. 1 (August 2009): 333–39, doi: 10.1097/AOG.0b013e3181ae9a47, http://www.ncbi.nlm.nih.gov/pubmed/19622995.

107. C. M. Furber et al., "Antenatal Interventions for Reducing Weight in Obese Women for Improving Pregnancy Outcome," *Cochrane Databases Systemic Reviews* (January 31, 2013), doi: 10.1002/14651858.CD009334.pub2, http://www.ncbi.nlm. nih.gov/pubmed/23440836.

108. Vireday, "Please Document Your Stories of Mistreatment"; Pamela Vireday, "Putting the Baby on a Diet Before It's Even Born," *The Well-Rounded Mama* (blog), October 9, 2008, accessed May 31, 2013, http://www.wellroundedmama.blogspot. com/2008/10/putting-baby-on-diet-before-its-even.html,; Pamela Vireday, "Bad Nutritional Advice to Pregnant Women," March 3, 2013, accessed May 31, 2013, http://www.wellroundedmama.blogspot.com/2013/03/bad-nutritional-advice-to -pregnant.html.

109. "Babies Given Anti-Obesity Drugs in the Womb," *Telegraph*, May 11, 2011, accessed May 28, 2013, http://www.telegraph.co.uk/health/healthnews/8505630/ Babies-given-anti-obesity-drugs-in-the-womb.html.

110. Lisa Collier Cool, "Unborn Babies Treated for Obesity in Womb," *Yahoo Health*, April 2, 2012, accessed May 29, 2013, http://health.yahoo.net/experts/ dayinhealth/should-unborn-babies-be-treated-obesity.

111. Shirley S. Wang, "Programming a Fetus for a Healthier Life," *Wall Street Journal*, July 5, 2011, accessed May 31, 2013, http://online.wsj.com/article/ SB10001424052702303763404576420240288155556.html.

112. J. Zheng, P. F. Shan, and W. Gu, "The Efficacy of Metformin in Pregnant Women with Polycystic Ovary Syndrome: A Meta-Analysis of Clinical Trials," *Journal of Endocrinological Investigation* (April 12, 2013), http://www.ncbi.nlm.nih .gov/pubmed/23580001.

113. T. M. Wensel, "Role of Metformin in the Treatment of Gestational Diabetes," *The Annals of Pharmacotherapy* 43, no. 5 (May 2009): 939–43, doi: 10.1345/ aph.1L562, http://www.ncbi.nlm.nih.gov/pubmed/19401478.

114. Puhl and Heuer, "Obesity Stigma."

115. Mike Adams, "Is Obesity during Pregnancy Child Abuse?," *NaturalNews.com*, July 19, 2004, accessed June 5, 2013, http://www.naturalnews.com/001415.html.

116. Elle, "Kindergartners, YOU'RE DOOMED!!!!."

117. Rachel Reilly, "Should Obese Women Have Weight-Loss Surgery Before Pregnancy to Prevent Their Children from Becoming Fat?," *Health Medicine Network*, May 28, 2013, accessed May 29, 2013, http://healthmedicinet.com/i/ should-obese-women-have-weight-loss-surgery-before-pregnancy-to-prevent-their -children-from-becoming-fat/.

118. Sauer, "Real America."

119. Pamela Vireday, "Gaining Weight in Pregnancy Means a Cesarean?," *The Well-Rounded Mama* (blog), October 19, 2010, accessed May 31, 2013. http://www .wellroundedmama.blogspot.com/2010/10/gaining-weight-in-pregnancy-means.html.

120. "Fat Women Only Have Babies Because We Can't Stop Them"; Adams, "Is Obesity during Pregnancy Child Abuse?"

3

10 Things You Can Do Right Now to Ease Concerns about Your Weight and Improve Your Health

Jon Robison

Given the focus on weight by the health establishment, the government, and the media, it is not surprising that so many people in this country are anxious about their weight and their health. And there certainly is no shortage of recommendations out there directing people to lose weight with this or that diet, lifestyle program, or eating regimen.

Unfortunately, the research over the last 25 years is quite clear. There is no evidence that any of these approaches result in long-term weight loss for the vast majority of people who engage in them. There are no exceptions, and none of the approaches (low fat, low calorie, low carb, etc.) work any better than any of the others.

Even more unfortunately however, this complete lack of evidence does not stop people from being seduced into trying to lose weight with the latest reincarnation of these approaches. Yet despite the huge time, money, and emotional investment, successful long-term weight loss is achieved by only a handful of people. The result is widespread confusion and anxiety about food and widespread weight cycling—people losing and regaining weight over and over again. Furthermore, the relentless pressure, particularly on women and children, to lose weight increases the likelihood of eating disorders, disordered eating, and body hatred.

Is there no solution to the weight-related struggles so many people are having? Is there nothing people can do to ease their concerns about weight and health? The good news is that there is indeed. By substituting a health-centered approach for the traditional weight-centered approach, you are promoting good health.[1]

The health-centered approach targets lifestyle factors such as physical activity, quality of diet, and stress. It is weight-neutral because it treats weight as an outcome of these factors combined with genetics and environment rather than as a direct target for treatment. While this differs substantially from the traditional wisdom about weight and health, please keep in mind that the traditional wisdom in this case is clearly not working or helping and is likely causing considerable harm.[2]

The following 10 suggestions, based on this health-centered approach, can go a long way toward helping people to ease the concerns about their weight, while at the same time improving their health and the quality of their lives. References for further reading on each suggestion can be found at the end of the chapter.

1. SAVE YOUR TIME AND MONEY

Don't spend another minute or another dime on anything (book, clinic, TV show, etc.) or anybody (doctor, dietitian, relative, talk show host, etc.) that even remotely suggests they will help you lose weight permanently.

Nothing in the health and medical fields has been proven more soundly, over and over again for as long a period of time, as the fact that focusing on weight loss is unlikely to lead to permanent weight loss and more likely to lead to weight cycling and weight gain. People who diet repeatedly over the years end up weighing more than they would have if they had never dieted. Weight cycling can make all the health problems weight loss supposedly helps (diabetes, hypertension, lipid abnormalities, etc.) worse.[3]

NOTE: If you are a health professional, read claims made by weight loss researchers with great care. The National Institutes of Health says five years should be considered long-term success for weight loss programs. Anything less should be viewed with suspicion. Just as importantly, be sure to check and see how many people started in the study and how many people's data were actually used in the final analysis. It is not unusual for weight loss studies to claim as a success a relatively small amount of weight loss in a small subset of the people who began the study. This is bad science at best.[4]

2. JUST SAY NO!

Do not use (or let anyone else use) your weight or body mass index or any other measurement of body size or composition as an indicator of health.

None of these has been shown to be strongly related to or predictive of health. People can be healthy at a wide range of weights, body mass indexes, body fat percentages, etc. Similarly, people with "normal" or "optimal" body composition measurements can have the same health problems that are often referred to as weight related.[5]

3. ASK FOR ANSWERS

If you have a health condition commonly considered to be "weight related" (the most likely candidates are hypertension, abnormal cholesterol, abnormal blood glucose) and a health professional recommends weight loss as a solution, ask her or him the following questions:

- What is the success rate of the approach you are suggesting? (What is the likelihood I will regain the weight I lose?)
- What is likely to happen to my health condition if I lose the weight and then regain it?
- Is there any way to treat this condition that does not involve a focus on weight loss? (How would you treat a thin person who had this condition?)

The answers given by your health professional to these questions should look something like:

- The success rate is no better than 5 percent, so it is quite likely that you will gain back all of the weight that you lost and perhaps a bit more.
- It is quite possible that your health issues (high blood pressure, diabetes, abnormal cholesterol, etc.) will get worse after you regain the weight.
- All of these conditions can be helped through lifestyle changes with little or no weight loss (a health-centered approach). The best treatment for a fat person for any of these conditions is the same treatment that would be recommended for a thin person.[6]

If you don't get something like these answers, consider seeking help elsewhere.

For the special case of diabetes, see the section at the end of the chapter.

4. USE YOUR IMAGINATION

If you do not have a health condition but you are worried that you will develop one if you don't make some lifestyle changes to lose weight, try the following:

- Imagine that you are, right now, at the weight that you believe will be healthier.

- Work out a plan (with a health professional if desired) of the kinds of lifestyle changes you think you might be able to sustain to remain healthy at that weight.
- Implement that plan, right now, at your current weight.

Be sure your plan does not include any type of externally determined caloric intake or food restriction, since these have been proven not to work for most people. Steps 5–8 below refer to the kinds of changes that are most likely to help prevent and ameliorate these so-called weight-related health conditions. They will also help your body to settle around its natural (genetically programmed) healthy weight.

5. CONSIDER MOVING YOUR BODY

If you are relatively sedentary and you think engaging in more physical activity would help you to be healthier, find ways to move your body that feel good to you.

The most up-to-date information on exercise is encouraging, especially for people who have been sedentary and have had difficulty trying to live up to the ever-changing, complicated and demanding exercise recommendations from the government and health establishment.[7]

For the vast majority of people, fitness is a much more important indicator of health than fatness.

- The greatest gains in health-related fitness are achieved when people go from being sedentary to getting even small amounts of physical activity.
- Physical activity does not have to be done all at once to achieve significant health benefits—three 10-minute periods of exercise are as good as one 30-minute period.
- All kinds of movement count, including walking, gardening, dancing, sports, and running after your kids.

6. DECLARE YOUR INDEPENDENCE

Don't let anyone (that's right—anyone!) tell you what or how much to eat to lose weight. Our bodies have wonderful, intricate mechanisms to help us to know how much to eat to maintain a healthy weight. No set of rules, guidelines, or regulations provided by experts can come close to the precision of the complex interactions among hunger, appetite, and satiety that naturally help us regulate our food intake and our weight if we pay attention to them. Ignoring these internal cues by following endless sets of external ones (Weight Watchers, Jenny Craig, The Food Pyramid, etc.) is likely to result in more rather than less disordered eating. A growing body of research suggests that adults and children who diet are more likely to gain extra weight as they get older than those who don't.[8]

7. LISTEN TO YOUR INTERNAL WISDOM

Learn to eat according to your internal signals; appetite, hunger, and satiety. By paying attention to these signals, you can avoid having to pay someone else to tell you what and how much to eat.[9]

For some people, eating can become a stand-in for other hungers that are not being satisfied. These may be related to a search for life balance, connection, or meaning and purpose. Sometimes, there may also be deep-seated struggles with depression, anxiety, and trauma that get played out with food. It is critical that these underlying issues be addressed. It is even more critical that no matter how much of a problem food and weight have become for an individual, with few exceptions, external food restriction will almost certainly cause more harm than good.

8. CONSIDER DR. ROBISON'S SIMPLIFIED DIETARY GUIDELINES

The original Four Food Groups were designed to help us to get the nutrition we need to grow and thrive. Over the years the Dietary Guidelines for Americans have become too complex, too prescriptive, and too focused on disease prevention and weight control.[10]

Some people may have a medical condition that requires them to eat or not eat particular foods. But for most people, the following guidelines can help establish the foundation for a nutritious diet while at the same time minimizing the constant worry about everything we put into our mouths—a seemingly ever-present stressor that is decidedly unhealthy! Here they are:

- Enjoy your food.
- Eat a wide variety of food.
- Pay attention to internal signals whenever you can.
- Share your food with someone who is needy—gratitude is deeply nourishing!

Bon appétit!

9. TAKE NOTICE OF WHAT REALLY MATTERS

Notice any changes that occur over time with this approach. Ask yourself:

- What health-related changes have I experienced?
- Do I feel differently about food?

- Do I feel differently about myself?
- Am I spending less time and energy worrying about my weight and what I am eating?

10. CELEBRATE

That's right! Congratulate yourself! It is very likely that you have:

- Ended your time on the frustrating rollercoaster that is dieting
- Increased your self-esteem and body image
- Taken charge of your eating by paying attention to your body instead of paying someone else to tell you what to do
- Helped your body settle near the weight it is genetically programmed to achieve
- Opened up potentially significant amounts of time and energy that you used to spend worrying and fretting about your weight and food
- Ameliorated or normalized any of the so-called weight-related health conditions you may have had whether or not you experienced any change in weight

THE "SPECIAL CASE" OF TYPE 2 DIABETES

But Dr. Robison, don't we need to recommend weight loss for people with type 2 diabetes? The answer to this question is a resounding "No!" Here is why:

- There is no evidence that weight loss interventions work for people with type 2 diabetes (most likely they work even less well than for the general weight loss-seeking population).
- Losing weight and then gaining it back can cause blood glucose problems to get worse. Since the vast majority of people will gain their weight back, this is a major issue.
- The good news is that research clearly demonstrates that problems with blood glucose can be helped greatly by using a health-centered approach without significant weight loss and even in people who gain body fat during the course of the study.[11]

Diabetes is a serious disease that causes great hardship and suffering for those who have it. However, the idea that we are currently experiencing an "epidemic" of diabetes has been oversold. According to the U.S. Centers for Disease Control, during the 1990s, when the "explosion" of overweight and obesity was said to occur, the most accurate data suggest only a small increase in the incidence of diabetes. Similarly, despite a good deal of fearmongering to the contrary, type 2 diabetes remains a rare occurrence in children. Statements to the contrary are often based on physicians' anecdotal reports or large phone interviews, neither of which can substitute for representative population data.

Because the concepts that thin equals healthy and weight loss equals better health are so deeply ingrained into the fabric of our culture, after examining this different approach people will often still ask this final question: if I do all of this will I lose weight? The answer to this question goes straight to the heart of the difference between the health-centered and weight-centered approaches. The answer is that, if people follow the suggestions outlined here, there are three and only three possibilities:

1. They will lose weight.
2. They will gain weight.
3. Their weight will not change.

What is wonderful about this answer, unlike almost any other answer related to this topic, is that it is undeniably scientific and unarguably true. If people are above their natural weight, they may lose some weight. If people are below their natural weight, they may gain. If people are close to their natural weight, they may stay the same. Which one of these outcomes will occur is often not predictable. What is predictable is that people will end up healthier and much less concerned about their weight and their health.

NOTES

1. Linda Bacon et al., "Size Acceptance and Intuitive Eating Improve Health for Obese, Female Chronic Dieters," *Journal of the American Dietetic Association* 105, no. 6 (2005): 929–36.

2. Linda Bacon and Lucy Aphramor, "Weight Science: Evaluating the Evidence for a Paradigm Shift," *Nutrition Journal* 10, no. 9 (2011), doi: 10.1186/1475-2891-10-9.

3. Traci Mann et al., "Medicare's Search for Effective Obesity Treatments," *American Psychologist* 62, no. 3 (2007): 220–33.

4. Lucy Aphramor, "Validity of Claims Made in Weight Management Research: A Narrative Review of Dietetic Articles," *Nutrition Journal* 9, no. 30 (2010), accessed January 6, 2014, http://www.nutritionj.com/content/9/1/30.

5. Dr. Keith Devlin, "Do You Believe in Fairies, Unicorns, or the BMI?," accessed January 6, 2014, http://www.maa.org/devlin/devlin_05_09.html; Rachel P. Wildman et al., "The Obese without Cardiometabolic Risk Factor Clustering and the Normal Weight with Cardiometabolic Risk Factor Clustering," *Archives of Internal Medicine* 168, no. 15 (2008): 1617–24.

6. Glenn Gaesser, *Big Fat Lies: The Truth about Your Weight and Your Health* (Carlsbad, CA: Gurze Books, 2002).

7. Glenn Gaesser, "Fatness, Fitness, and Health: A Closer Look at the Evidence," *WELCOA, Absolute Advantage* 5, no. 3 (2006): 18–21; Paul A. McAuley and Steven Blair, "Obesity Paradoxes," *Journal of Sports Sciences* 29, no. 8 (2011): 773–82.

8. Dianne Neumark-Sztainer et al., "Dieting and Unhealthy Weight Control Behaviors during Adolescence: Associations with 10-Year Changes in Body Mass Index," *Journal of Adolescent Health* 50 (2012): 80–86.

9. Ellyn Satter, *Secrets of Feeding a Healthy Family* (Madison, WI: Kelcy Press, 2008); Evelyn Tribole and Elyse Resch, *Intuitive Eating: A Revolutionary Program That Works*, 2nd ed. (New York: St. Martin's Griffin, 2010).

10. Ellyn Satter, "Dietary Guidelines and Food Guide Pyramid Incapacitate Consumers and Contribute to Distorted Eating Attitudes and Behaviors," accessed January 6, 2014, http://www.ellynsatter.com/resources.jsp.

11. Linda Bacon and Judith Matz, "Intuitive Eating: Enjoy Your Food, Respect Your Body," *Diabetes Self-Management* (November/December 2010): 45–51.

4

Making Healthy Eating a Reality through Size Acceptance and Intuitive Eating

Marsha Hudnall

Ask the average person these days to define healthy eating and you'll likely hear a recitation of diet rules. Such and such food is "good"; another kind of food is "bad." The bad foods are "fattening" and if you eat any, you've ruined any attempt at healthy eating that day. This is another indication of diet thinking at work—if you "blow it" one day, you start again the next day, week, month, after a period of overindulgence on "forbidden" foods. Eating reasonably the next time you eat isn't even considered.

While restricting eating in an attempt to control body size is reported as far back as 1,000 years ago, the current popularity of weight loss diets appears to have begun to take hold in the early 1960s, evidenced by the appearance of Metrecal, one of the first liquid diet products produced specifically for weight loss. Since then, countless diets have appeared on the scene, many tied to manufactured food products, but all dictating specific guidelines for what, when, and how much to eat in order to lose weight.

Even though dieting has become synonymous with effective weight management in the average person's mind, research clearly shows that the practice leads people in the exact opposite direction. Most people end up gaining weight instead of losing it. Further, dieting is recognized as a factor in the development of eating disorders and disordered eating behaviors, which have increased among those living in a Western culture in recent years. Eating disorder behaviors, which include emotional overeating behaviors such as binge eating, have been documented in people of all ages, genders, ethnic minority groups, and levels of education and income. Indeed, binge eating disorder is the most common eating disorder in the United States, and an estimated 3.5 percent of women, 2 percent of men, and 30 to 40 percent of those seeking weight loss treatments can be clinically diagnosed with binge eating disorder.[1]

A recent study of more than 35,000 people found strong associations between dieting and emotional eating.[2]

In this chapter, I take a step back to look at a definition of healthy eating that is not based on attempts to control body size, looking through the lens of eating in a way that is evolutionarily supportive of health and well-being. In today's parlance, that way is called intuitive eating, e.g., eating according to internal cues that do not depend on rules or other external guidelines but instead have developed over the course of human evolution to guide eating for well-being. This will be explored as a prelude to a discussion of how size acceptance is critical in order for a person to eat intuitively to achieve healthy eating and wellness goals, as well as insight into the process of reconnecting with internal cues for eating and the outcomes that a person can expect from that process.

EATING WELL DEFINED

A quick Internet search finds eating well defined in a variety of ways that reflect the current high interest in health and wellness as well as concern over technological developments that have affected the production and nutritional quality of the food supply.

Ultimately, however, the popular notion of eating well is primarily dependent on nutrition. Whole foods, that is, foods that are as close to their natural state as possible and therefore contain the natural mix and amounts of nutrients that are important to human health, are considered the foundation of eating well. Eating a variety of whole foods is also key in order to get a wide mix of nutrients, and various groupings of foods have been devised over the years to guide eating a healthy mix of foods. Currently, these groups include vegetables and fruits, grains, and protein foods such as meat, fish, poultry, eggs, legumes, and dairy foods.

Given the vast number of foods available today that do not qualify as whole foods yet are commonly eaten for pleasure, such as snack foods like chips, candies, and the like, many nutritionists encourage a gentle application of rational thinking when it comes to choosing what to eat. In the book *Intuitive Eating*, which popularized the term "intuitive eating," coauthors Evelyn Tribole, RD, and Elyse Resch, RD, call this rational thinking "gentle nutrition." Table 4.1 lists the principles of intuitive eating according to Tribole and Resch's book; the 10th principle focuses on the fact that "perfect eating" isn't necessary to achieve nutrition and health goals, alluding to the fact that pleasure may be as important as nutrition when it comes to eating. Pleasure creates a relaxation response that supports the improved digestion, absorption, and metabolism of the food we eat.[3]

TABLE 4.1   10 Principles of Intuitive Eating

1. Reject the Diet Mentality

Throw out the diet books and magazine articles that offer you false hope of losing weight quickly, easily, and permanently. Get angry at the lies that have led you to feel as if you were a failure every time a new diet stopped working and you gained back all of the weight. If you allow even one small hope to linger that a new and better diet might be lurking around the corner, it will prevent you from being free to rediscover intuitive eating.

2. Honor Your Hunger

Keep your body biologically fed with adequate energy and carbohydrates. Otherwise you can trigger a primal drive to overeat. Once you reach the moment of excessive hunger, all intentions of moderate, conscious eating are fleeting and irrelevant. Learning to honor this first biological signal sets the stage for rebuilding trust with yourself and food.

3. Make Peace with Food

Call a truce, stop the food fight! Give yourself unconditional permission to eat. If you tell yourself that you can't or shouldn't have a particular food, it can lead to intense feelings of deprivation that build into uncontrollable cravings and, often, bingeing, When you finally "give in" to your forbidden food, eating will be experienced with such intensity that it usually results in Last Supper overeating, and overwhelming guilt.

4. Challenge the Food Police

Scream a loud "NO" to thoughts in your head that declare you're "good" for eating minimal calories or "bad" because you ate a piece of chocolate cake. The Food Police monitor the unreasonable rules that dieting has created. The police station is housed deep in your psyche, and its loudspeaker shouts negative barbs, hopeless phrases, and guilt-provoking indictments. Chasing the Food Police away is a critical step in returning to intuitive eating.

5. Respect Your Fullness

Listen for the body signals that tell you that you are no longer hungry. Observe the signs that show that you're comfortably full. Pause in the middle of a meal or food and ask yourself how the food tastes and what your current fullness level is.

6. Discover the Satisfaction Factor

The Japanese have the wisdom to promote pleasure as one of their goals of healthy living. In our fury to be thin and healthy, we often overlook one of the most basic gifts of existence—the pleasure and satisfaction that can be found in the eating experience. When you eat what you really want, in an environment that is inviting and conducive, the pleasure you derive will be a powerful force in helping you feel satisfied and content. By providing this experience for yourself, you will find that it takes much less food to decide you've had "enough."

7. Honor Your Feelings without Using Food

Find ways to comfort, nurture, distract, and resolve your issues without using food. Anxiety, loneliness, boredom, and anger are emotions we all experience throughout life.

(*continued*)

TABLE 4.1 (Continued)

Each has its own trigger, and each has its own appeasement. Food won't fix any of these feelings. It may comfort for the short term, distract from the pain, or even numb you into a food hangover. But food won't solve the problem. If anything, eating for an emotional hunger will only make you feel worse in the long run. You'll ultimately have to deal with the source of the emotion, as well as the discomfort of overeating.

8. Respect Your Body

Accept your genetic blueprint. Just as a person with a shoe size of 8 would not expect to realistically squeeze into a size 6, it is equally as futile (and uncomfortable) to have the same expectation with body size. But mostly, respect your body so you can feel better about who you are. It's hard to reject the diet mentality if you are unrealistic and overly critical about your body shape.

9. Exercise—Feel the Difference

Forget militant exercise. Just get active and feel the difference. Shift your focus to how it feels to move your body, rather than the calorie-burning effect of exercise. If you focus on how you feel from working out, such as energized, it can make the difference between rolling out of bed for a brisk morning walk or hitting the snooze alarm. If when you wake up your only goal is to lose weight, it's usually not a motivating factor in that moment of time.

10. Honor Your Health—Gentle Nutrition

Make food choices that honor your health and taste buds while making you feel well. Remember that you don't have to eat a perfect diet to be healthy. You will not suddenly get a nutrient deficiency or gain weight from one snack, one meal, or one day of eating. It's what you eat consistently over time that matters; progress not perfection is what counts.

Note: See http://www.intuitiveeating.org/content/10-principles-intuitive-eating.

Even though it is key, the concept of eating for pleasure is an important but much-ignored component of eating well. At least it's much ignored these days, due in large part to the fundamental tenet of most weight loss diets that foods high in fat, sugar, and salt are instrumental in weight struggles and therefore must be eliminated or eaten rarely. Yet fat, sugar, and salt add significant flavor to foods and can be part of healthy eating when used in moderation.

Moderation, however, has become a stand-in word for restriction in the minds of many. In diet lingo, advice to eat moderately is often interpreted as advice to restrict what and how much you eat. Rebecca Scritchfield, registered dietitian and intuitive-eating coach, compares the true meaning of both words: "Moderation means that each person is responsible for eating in a way that feels pleasurable and calm vs. something they think they should be ashamed of or sneak and hide," says Scritchfield. "It also means being able to pay enough attention to what you're doing to know that food doesn't feel good when you overeat it. Restriction means setting strict rules, and labeling foods as good/allowed and bad/not allowed. For example telling your kids that cookies are not allowed in the house because they're bad for you. Kids are born intuitive eaters that recognize when they've eaten too much."[4]

So the concept of moderation allows for the inclusion of foods rich in fat, sugar, and salt in a healthy eating plan. And it bears repeating that pleasure is a key component in eating well. Taste repeatedly ranks first on surveys of why people choose the foods they do, meaning that enjoyment of what we eat is key to us continuing to eat it. On-again, off-again efforts at "healthy eating" characterize weight loss diets because of one simple truth: if we don't enjoy something, it's not easy to keep doing it. Pleasure is an inherent motivator, and anyone attempting to change a behavior is wise to figure out how to find the fun in the target behavior.

Finally, when we don't enjoy something, we also run the risk of causing stress, which is a well-known outcome of dieting for weight loss. Stress negatively affects the digestion, absorption, and metabolism of foods and therefore has the potential to diminish the nutritional benefit derived from foods. Conversely, enjoyment is a great way to de-stress, which underscores the value of pleasure in eating well.

It's worthwhile to note here that a similar approach can be taken toward engaging in regular physical activity, another key aspect of healthy living. Weight loss plans have traditionally tied physical activity to burning calories, which then ends up as a form of punishment for eating and, hence, another on-again, off-again endeavor for many who struggle with eating and weight. In reality, physical activity plays important roles in health in a variety of ways, including reducing stress and the production of hormones that support health. It also helps "reconnect the head to the body"—chronic dieters and emotional eaters often end up "living from the neck up," worrying about what they eat with little awareness of how it makes them feel. Physical activity supports the efficient and effective operation of the internal cues that can guide eating.

THE IMPORTANCE OF SIZE ACCEPTANCE TO EATING WELL

Intuitive eating (and exercise), then, paves the way to true healthy eating, guided by an individual's innate knowledge of what his or her body needs at any one moment. Concern about body size impacts a person's ability to eat intuitively much like restriction impacts a person's ability to eat moderately. Because of the dieting-induced link between what we eat and the concern about body size that is deeply embedded in the popular psyche, concern about body size acts as a form of restriction. When they worry about their weight, people who don't eat intuitively also worry about what and how much they eat, leading to sporadic attempts at "healthy eating" that end up as an eating pattern that is far different from the true definition of the term.

In a groundbreaking randomized clinical trial, PhD nutritionist Linda Bacon found that size acceptance and intuitive eating were key to sustainable lifestyle behavior change, including healthy eating.[5] Women who took part in a Health at Every Size treatment group showed significant and sustained improvements in health measures that are affected by eating patterns, such as blood cholesterol and blood pressure levels, as compared to those who those who were treated with a standard diet protocol. This study was the first to show that decreasing the focus on weight loss as part of health improvement efforts better supports the ability to achieve health goals.

Two of the five principles that make up the Health at Every Size approach to health and wellness involve size acceptance and intuitive eating; accepting and respecting the diversity of body sizes and shapes, and eating in a manner that balances individual nutritional needs, hunger, satiety, appetite, and pleasure. Subsequent research has confirmed Bacon's findings that a Health at Every Size approach is "associated with statistically and clinically relevant improvements in physiological measures (e.g., blood pressure, blood lipids), health behaviors (e.g., physical activity, eating disorder pathology) and psychosocial outcomes (e.g., mood, self-esteem, body image)."[6]

MOVING TO INTUITIVE EATING

While intuitive eating is a natural process of the body, the term is frequently used to describe approaches that reeducate people about how to eat normally, e.g., without following diet rules. The most well known of those approaches is the book *Intuitive Eating*, referenced above. The eighth principle of their approach identifies size acceptance as fundamental to its success (Table 4.1).

Other authors offer different approaches with different names but still incorporate the theme of using the body's natural cues to guide eating, supported by an acceptance of natural body size. For example, Ellyn Satter's eating competence model builds on natural tendencies toward food to support health and well-being. Satter describes how she came to develop her model. "I consistently found prescriptive dietary interventions to undermine my patients' foodways, to destroy their ability to intuitively regulate food intake, to worsen their nutritional status and to spoil their attitudes about eating."[7] Satter has long identified weight loss diets as the type of prescriptive dietary intervention that does not support healthy eating.

Other names used to describe a natural way of eating include attuned eating, conscious eating, and mindful eating.

It is important to note that successfully moving from a weight-loss-centered approach to eating to an approach that heeds internal cues is a process for many. Years of sporadic dieting interspersed with prolonged periods of eating "forbidden" foods of low nutrient quality can result in physiologic imbalances that mean the body's natural cues may not work properly at first. In addition, from a psychological perspective, fear about eating and weight leads to a distrust of the body's cues. Often, efforts may need to focus first on learning to recognize and trust the body's cues. At Green Mountain at Fox Run, my women's health retreat that pioneered the nondiet approach to healthy living, we use a structured approach to help put the body back into balance physiologically and also provide exposure to feared foods to enable a successful encounter with such foods, e.g., eating them without overeating them. As people become more confident and trusting of their bodies' cues, they can return to intuitive eating as second nature: it's not something they need to spend time thinking about—it's just how they eat.

SIZE ACCEPTANCE AND SUCCESS

The following stories from real women illustrate the change that intuitive eating coupled with size acceptance can produce in a person's relationship with food and ability to eat more healthfully.

Trudi was introduced to intuitive eating and size acceptance at Green Mountain. She describes her journey to gaining peace with her eating and her weight through this approach. She explained:

> Food almost never represented nutrition to me nor did I associate it with good health. Food and the act of eating were sometimes social, but mostly I consumed food in response to every emotion possible—happiness, sadness, anger, frustration, boredom, anxiety, etc.
>
> Dieting contributed to my struggle with emotional overeating. After an episode of overeating, I would be upset and punish myself with yet more food. Then, of course, I would tell myself that the diet begins again tomorrow (or Monday, or after the holiday, or when the company leaves, or on the first of the month, well, you get the idea!). Until then, though, I would eat as though it was going to be my last meal.
>
> During times of rigid dieting, I treated food as the enemy and really restricted both my intake as well as my food choices. Body weight was always on my mind. I liked myself only in accordance with what the number on the scale read. Even when I achieved a weight goal, it was never good enough. I always saw the fat girl in the mirror. I had a dietitian once tell me that I had anorexic tendencies. Me? Surely, you jest. At the time I took that comment as the highest form of flattery!
>
> I lived on the weight-loss-&-gain-it-back roller coaster. Through very rigid and restrictive eating, I was almost always able to lose weight, but keeping it off for any length of time seemed impossible. My fitness goals

were equally stringent. I walked every day for two hours after work—no matter what the temperature or weather conditions were. Once I was out in a thunderstorm with lots of lightning and my dad drove around until he found me and insisted I ride home with him. I refused; he was not happy. Another time I was out in below zero temperatures walking my usual route and a neighbor stopped and offered me a ride home. Again, I refused. After completing my mandatory two-hour walk, I would then come home and ride my stationary bike for one hour. There were times that I would only stop if I literally fell off of the bike due to fatigue. My calf muscles cramped on me frequently, and often times when I was driving.

In retrospect it is surprising how many years I lived this way. The time finally came when my lifestyle had to change (due to marriage), and the weight piled back on, and the more I gained, the more I punished myself with food. I felt frustrated and angry that I was allowing this to happen to me, and that just led to more of the same destructive behavior.

At one point I resorted to dangerous weight loss methods including taking ephedra. It gave me so much energy and I felt so good, it couldn't possibly be harmful. Until I developed heart palpitations and had to stop using it. I had lost 40+ pounds and looked good, but at what cost?

My relationship with food, exercise and my body began to change when I attended the program at Green Mountain at Fox Run. I am now a more mindful and intuitive eater. I learned food is not the enemy. It provides me with the energy I need to do the things I want and need to do each and every day, and it's also something I enjoy. I began experimenting with how different foods make me feel and discovered the types of food that give me sustained energy and that truly satisfy my taste buds

I am definitely a more mindful and intuitive eater now. I practice moderation instead of abstinence and without feelings of guilt. I try to wait for hunger signals, be thoughtful about my food selection, focus on my food as I eat, and most importantly I am working on self acceptance, especially as it relates to my size.

I don't have it all figured out yet, but it feels like I'm on the right path. I am well on my way to learning how to substitute activities other than eating to deal with stress, sadness, boredom, frustration and all of the other reasons I ate other than the real reason to eat – hunger. I am learning how to recognize real, honest-to-goodness hunger. It's been a long, long time since I've been able to do that.

It certainly is an on-going process—a journey—but I do feel that what I took home from Green Mountain has helped me to become a person I like a whole lot better than I did previously. I feel like my commitment to personal growth and change in this area is a form of respect for myself.

Jill's relationship with food changed dramatically after moving to size acceptance and intuitive eating. She describes the evolving nature of that relationship in this post that first appeared on Green Mountain's blog *A Weight Lifted*. Jill blogs regularly at *Eating as a Path to Yoga*. She said:

> Most recently, I've been working on sitting with the uncomfortable feelings of loss, the loss of a very dear friend. You may have met her. Her name is Food.
>
> The first time there was a rift in our relationship is when I stopped binge eating. I had to sit with very extreme feelings in order not to binge. I had to learn to take care of myself in a new way. That way was creating new neural pathways, or habits, so that I didn't always turn to my friend, Food.
>
> I also found other healthy friends such as Yoga, Journaling, & Sleep. Balance is important in friendships. You don't want to be dependent upon just one person. You can become too entwined. It's good to let others in as well, to give you perspective.
>
> What I'm working on now with Food, however, is learning to stop at the point of satisfaction. I want to take care of my body. But filling it up with food it no longer needs isn't working for me from a self-care standpoint or making me feel well. More importantly, it isn't balanced.
>
> Food and I can be friends, but we just can't be codependent. I'm learning to sit with the feelings of being sad that it is time to stop eating. Unlike different friends, such alcohol & drugs, I can't live without food. It will always be part of my life. We may not be best friends, but we will still see each other in the kitchen, at book club, or even at the grocery store.
>
> Our relationship with each other is evolving to a healthier place. When I grieve the loss of my friend, I can still have hope that I will see her again. Food isn't like the grandma you see once a year. You can see her as many times in a day that you choose. You are in charge of what your relationship will be. Some days you may see her more often than others. Friendship is like that.

Annabel describes her experience with giving up dieting, accepting her body, and what it has meant to her eating, her health, and her well-being. She also shares tips for getting on the path to a diet-free life. This also appeared on *A Weight Lifted*. Annabel blogs regularly at *Feed Me I'm Cranky*. She shared:

Last year, I did something unheard of: I gave up dieting. This may not seem like a big deal, but in a society that fosters body-shame backed by a $60B weight-loss industry, it IS a big deal.

I'm not going to give you the false impression that giving up dieting was easy. In fact, giving up the hope, and desire for, weight loss has been harder—for me—than losing weight itself. So why bother? If I can lose weight, shouldn't I? Shouldn't I at least try?

No. It's a slippery slope and I'll tell you why: If you're not "good enough" now, you'll never be. Dieting is not a means to self-acceptance; in fact, dieting is the quickest way to give yourself a potentially dangerous complex. You'll notice that you start thinking of yourself as "good" and "worthy" when you eat less and weigh less and "bad" and "unworthy" when you eat more or weigh more. Worse—you'll begin this thing that I call a "weight-centered contingency plan," i.e. everything in life from travel plans to pursuing a romantic interest to wearing certain cuts of dresses will be put on hold until you reach a certain weight. The problem is, once you get on this contingency plan, the end goal becomes fluid. You'll find that if your goal weight was x and you reach it, a new lower weight goal will probably replace it.

So, you may be wondering, how does one give up dieting? The most helpful thing for me to do when I decided to stop dieting was to ask myself critical questions. I'm going to list some of them below, in bold, with the answers I came up with after truly digging deep. You'll see that by asking these questions I was able to get past some of the falsities and fears that were embedded in my head. I hope that this exercise will help any of you who are dieting and would rather make peace with your body:

- **How is dieting working for you?** It depends on what we mean by "dieting." Dieting itself has not helped me get healthy; becoming curious and empowered about nutrition and fitness along with a host of other things, like stability in my home life and finances, mental work on self-perception, etc., have worked in unison to make me healthier. Dieting is not sustainable because it requires that I see food as a means to weight loss/weight maintenance rather than the complex and wonderful source of energy that it is. In other words, I'll just diet myself into poor physical and mental health if I'm always gauging how and what I eat based on my weight.
- **Do you want to do this for the rest of your life?** Do I want to count, measure and restrict for the rest of my life? No way! My body is going to continue to change as I grow older, potentially have kids, potentially get sick or injured, as my schedule changes, as my interests change, etc. I have a world to conquer and so many awesome things to achieve—a certain size

or weight is not one of them because there is no intrinsic value there! In other words, the only "value" I get from weight loss in and of itself is value that society bestows upon me for getting closer to the mainstream conventional standard of beauty, which is, arguably, unobtainable in a healthful way. The way to free yourself from the "standard" of beauty is not to try complying with it, but rather to identify it for what it is: oppressive, unrealistic and shallow.

- How important is your weight really? It's not the sole determinant of my health, or even a good proxy for my health. Weight is correlated to health, but not causally related. Weight is correlated to health, just like where you live, who your family is, how much money you make, whether you went to college, what your job is, etc., is correlated to health. If we are looking outside of health, then, yes, we see that being thin (and thin-pretty) carries a tremendous real-world value in our society. We also see that people are continually stigmatized and discriminated based on weight. I would be lying to say that weight does not/cannot dramatically affect your life. However, just because society places value (and restricts rights) based on weight does not make it right and does not mean that the answer to discrimination is attempted compliance! The truth of the matter is that healthful habits make us healthy.[8] Even Michelle Obama recently said that health is "not about size or weight." Way to go, FLOTUS!

- What do you really want and can you get it by focusing outside of your weight? I really want to love myself, and my body, without any contingencies, including weight-based contingencies. I want to love and relish in my body throughout all of its stages. I want to treat myself well and be well. I actually have to focus outside of my weight to achieve these things.

- Can dieting actually be harmful? Dieting IS harmful. When dieting, I have to ignore my biological instincts, hunger and satiation cues. When dieting, I stop listening to what my body craves. When weight is the focus, I see exercise as punishment for eating or as a "necessary evil." Dieting forces me to detach from my body. Dieting means my energy and focus is on my weight rather than on doing fun, positive and wonderful things for and in this world. Dieting makes me angry, tired, and resentful. It takes the enjoyment out of food. It makes eating a stress-based activity. It makes me see food as the enemy rather than as a life-giving source that is my ALLY in making me healthy.

- What's holding you back from quitting dieting? Fear. If I stop dieting, I will gain weight. Hm. But will I? (NO, not necessarily. If we are eating mindfully, our body gets to its optimal and healthy size.) Is living a fear-based life the path you want to take for the long haul? No. I would rather do the work now to learn to love my body in all its stages than to spend the rest of my life dieting.

- What's the worst that can happen if you stop dieting? I could gain weight. Is that a valid a concern? All concerns are valid because you feel them, but should we reframe this? Yes. Maybe you should start asking, "What GREAT things would happen if I stopped dieting?" The benefits blow the potential, and fallacious, cons out of the water.
- Is this a diet? It's not a "lifestyle change" if it has weight as a measure of "success." If weight is a measure, it's a diet (don't fool yourself!).

I Gave Up Dieting; You Can, Too

Are you ready to stop dieting? Here are three quick ways to get on the path to a diet-free life:

1. Answer all of the critical questions above honestly. Write down your answers and refer to them whenever you feel the urge to go on a "spring cleanse" or the urge to get "bikini ready" (p.s. you ARE biking ready!)
2. Fill your brain with allies. Read weight-neutral books, size acceptance books and Health At Every Size® books (some of my favorites include If Not Dieting Then What?[9], What's Wrong with Fat?[10] And Health at Every Size: The Surprising Truth about Your Weight[11] and size-acceptance blogs like Dances with Fat[12] Fit and Feminist[13] and Deah Schwartz[14] (there are SO many good ones!).
3. Remember that feeling shame in your body will never lead you to good health or a slimmer figure. Remember that there is a $60B industry out there that is doing everything it can to make you hate yourself so that you can pay them for a "solution" that doesn't exist (in other words, if anyone had a true and sustainable solution for weight loss, the industry wouldn't be worth $60B and there would be no fat people).

NOTES

1. Binge Eating Disorder Association, http://www.bedaonline.com.

2. Peneau et al., "Sex and Dieting Modify the Association between Emotional Eating and Weight Status," *The American Journal of Clinical Nutrition* 97, no. 6 (June 2013): 1307–13.

3. http://umm.edu/health/medical/reports/articles/stress.

4. Rebecca Scritchfield, http://rebeccascritchfield.wordpress.com/2013/06/06/new-research-released-about-food-restriction-pressure-and-kids/ accessed 5/19/14

5. L. Bacon et al., "Size Acceptance and Intuitive Eating Improve Health for Obese, Female Chronic Dieters," *Journal of the American Dietetic Association* 105 (2005): 929–36.

6. L. Bacon and L. Aphramor, "Weight Science: Evaluating the Evidence for a Paradigm Shift," *Nutrition Journal* 10, no. 69 (2011), doi: 10.1186 /1475-2891-10-9.

7. http://www.ellynsatter.com/november-16-2007-family-meals-focus-21-eating-competence-i-119.html.

8. See E. M. Matheson et al., "Healthy Lifestyle Habits and Mortality in Overweight and Obese Individuals," *Journal of the American Board of Family Medicine* 25, no. 1 (January–February 2012: 9–15, http://www.jabfm.org/content/25/1/9.abstract?etoc; M. Wei et al., "Relationship between Low Cardiorespiratory Fitness and Mortality in Normal-Weight, Overweight, and Obese Men," *Journal of the American Medical Association* 282, no. 16 (October 27, 1999):1547–53, http://www.ncbi.nlm.nih.gov/pubmed/10546694; D. L. Chong, "Cardiorespiratory Fitness, Body Composition, and All-Cause and Cardiovascular Disease Mortality in Men," *The American Journal of Clinical Nutrition* 69, no. 3 (March 1999): 373–80, http://ajcn.nutrition.org/content/69/3/373.full.

9. Rick Kausman, "If Not Dieting, Then What?," http://www.ifnotdieting.com.au/cpa/htm/htm_store_product_view.asp?id=11.

10. A. C. Saguy, *What's Wrong with Fat?* (New York: Oxford University Press, 2013).

11. L. Bacon, *Health at Every Size: The Surprising Truth about Your Weight* (Dallas, TX: BenBella Books, 2008, 2010).

12. http://danceswithfat.wordpress.com/.

13. http://fitandfeminist.wordpress.com/.

14. http://www.drdeah.com/blog/.

5

All the Way from B(lame) to A(cceptance): Diabetes, Health, and Fat Activism

Jennifer Lee

As an academic who is writing about fat within the multidisciplinary and interdisciplinary field of fat studies, I often feel that I am writing for a broader audience than some academics do within other disciplines. If I was to play a game of word association, what word do you think of upon reading these words: diabetes, heart disease, stroke, gluttonous, lazy, and undisciplined? Whether you believe the associations between these words and "obesity" or "overweight" or "fat," it is likely that most readers know the link is often made between those words. I am working in a fraught and contentious research area, where it seems nearly everyone in our Western culture has a stake, everyone has an opinion—some based on research, some based on prejudice, and some based on the proliferation of inadequate scientific research with inappropriate controls or even deliberately skewed hypotheses. There is often underlying hostility for academics working in the fat studies field, from other disciplines and sometimes from the institutions we work for. There is a vested interest in obesity research funding at universities and in the continued narrative that obesity is unhealthy and bad and has reached epidemic proportions.[1]

Sometimes when I write about being fat I cut out large chunks of writing about peripheral issues—believing that, as most writers do, I am "getting off track." When I began writing this chapter about diabetes, fat, and fat activism, I decided I wanted to leave these other influencing aspects in the piece. Autoethnographic academic writing is becoming more common, especially in the humanities, as it allows a writer to declare and explore her personal experiences and contextualize her position—whether she is developing an explicit and singular argument, or, as I have done here, exploring the issues surrounding being fat, a fat activist, and someone recently diagnosed with a typical "fat" disease—type 2 diabetes.

This chapter tells the story of a particular time in my life and, in academic fashion, refers to evidence and other perspectives where it is really needed to contextualize.

I am a fat woman and I was diagnosed with type 2 diabetes about two years ago. I am going to tell the stories that surround the diagnosis, as they shed light on my experience as a fat woman. In March 2010, I started in my first full-time ongoing academic position in the field of creative writing (the Australian equivalent of a tenured position). I got this job after working toward it with 10 years of casual academic work—and it was my dream job. When I began the job, my partner and I had been discussing when we should try to conceive a child. We had come close to starting the year before, but when I lost a part-time contract position at a different university, I focused on finding work instead.

The new academic job took over my life—I worked 12-hour days five days a week and 7-hour days on weekends. I am not a workaholic, but I am also not great at cutting corners. My social life, relationships, sense of self, level of exercise, sleeping patterns, and anxiety levels were all severely affected. We delayed attempting to have a child. The creeping, dark thought that maybe this wasn't my dream job after all surfaced. I had studied for 11 years and worked part-time in academia for a decade, living hand-to-mouth, and this "dream" job was almost too much for me. Because it was a dream job and I was told that 70 people went for the position, I convinced myself, over and over, to stick it out. There were great things about it too. In fact the job reminded me of a passionate relationship where you fight all the time—you love the job/lover, you cling onto it, you desperately want it to work, there are short but brilliant highs, but it exhausts you and leaves you with little energy for anything else in your life. Without an even-keeled supportive and giving partner who is fine in a nontraditional male role, I doubt I would have made it through those first three years in the job.

Along with the difficulties of overwork, a senior colleague I had spoken to about fat prejudice sent me a call for papers for a Sydney Fat Studies conference, organized by Dr. Samantha Murray from Macquarie University. I didn't feel ready to write a paper in the field, as that was the first I had heard about fat studies. But as a creative writer and arts event organizer, I secured funding from my department at the university and contacted the conference about organizing a reading and performance event. I teamed up with a Sydney group, Fat Femme Front, who curated the art exhibition for the conference. We had fat academics, writers, and artists performing poetry, memoir, fiction, stand-up comedy, all surrounded by fat art. It was the first time I had been in a fat acceptance space, and the audience shed tears at times, as did I. The camaraderie and support was like nothing I had experienced before. I once organized an event called "Femme Fever," for femme queer women, the first one that the Melbourne queer festival, Midsumma, had hosted, and that comes a close second. In both cases, a huge sold-out audience came together to say things that had not been said out in the open, to peel back the layers of taboo in our culture.

At that conference I met fat activists like Dr. Samantha Murray, Dr. Cat Pausé, Jackie Wykes, Dr. Charlotte Cooper, and Kelli Jean Drinkwater. At the time I didn't realize just how amazing it was to meet these women because I was too amazed by the content I was hearing and because I hadn't yet done the reading in the field. It was life changing and, while I had done years of work to shed a dieting and binge eating cycle through a moderate mindful-eating program, I had not yet understood how fat acceptance, how love and care of the body, worked. Not until I was surrounded by other fat women (and a few men) who identified as fat activists, fat artists, fat academics.

I read so many books and articles so fast after that conference, from *The Fat Female Body*[2] to *The Fat Studies Reader*[3] to *Health at Every Size*.[4] Jackie Wykes started a Melbourne chapter of Aquaporko, the fat synchronized swim team that Kelli Jean Drinkwater had started in Sydney and taken to the Sydney queer festival, Mardi Gras. I went to a few sessions of Aquaporko and learned how to do backflips and enjoyed the coffee-and-cake sessions afterward, even when a group of us were harassed by men who yelled "go on a diet" at us. The health rhetoric had infiltrated street harassment. Fat activity in Melbourne increased after the conference—there were fat clothes swaps, fat fashion parades, fat burlesque, and briefly I ran a fat studies reading group.

Then six months later I went to my general practitioner complaining of exhaustion, and she ran blood tests and found that my HBA1C, which measures glucose in the blood across the previous three months, was 6.5, which is in diabetic range. I knew my grandmother and uncle on my mum's side and my grandfather on my father's side were all diabetics, but they hadn't been early onset, or so I originally thought.

I avoided doctors for the first year after this, for fear of fat shaming. When I went to a dietitian (in Australia we have a public health system so, unless you opt to pay out of your own pocket, you are allocated to a medical professional) I was fat shamed badly; it triggered some negative thinking about food, and some previous eating disorder issues arose again. It took me several months to move on from her judgment. I then returned and paid for a Health at Every Size dietitian privately, who gave me some good advice.

I was referred to a good endocrinologist (who listens to me and doesn't discuss weight with me), but I've had some trouble with aspects of diabetes management that seem to be hooking back into eating disorder territory. What I mean is, in my twenties I went on extreme diets; did lots of calorie counting, banning of high-fat foods, weighing, and recording food; and experienced all that guilt associated with food. Then, after I had psychological treatment for binge eating disorder, I had several years of feeling more relaxed around food (but still some issues around wanting to lose weight) and then, in 2010, I had about six months of fat acceptance and being relaxed around food before I was diagnosed with diabetes. A year after I was diagnosed I followed medical advice and did more exercise, worked with weights, tried to eat more low-glycemic index foods, and I had to eat more often (every three hours). That made no difference to my blood sugar levels—absolutely no difference. Diabetics are often told that if we eat well and exercise, our blood sugar will improve, but mine didn't. I manage my anxiety and depression (untreated anxiety since I was about 5 years old, until I was about 30 years old), but I began to wonder what effect that has.

I'm struggling with the lack of control I have over my blood sugar—it seems like I can't "improve" my blood sugar numbers. I have also avoided checking my blood sugar several times a day, as when the numbers are too high, it triggers similar emotions to when I weighed myself. I think, "What have I eaten?"; "What have I done wrong?"; "What can I do better?"—all similar guilt-inducing thoughts I had when I used to weigh myself and hadn't lost weight. I struggle with feeling like a failure, and my body feels like a failure as well. What I see as obsessive measurement, recording, striving to achieve something through eating well and exercising—it's like my brain doesn't know the difference between why I'm engaging in these behaviors now and why I used to. The "monitoring" of my food intake is something I thought I could let go of, and now I feel trapped, back in that space.

Now that I want to try to conceive and become pregnant, I have to measure my blood much more often—four or five times a day—and I've been put on insulin, to take before I go to bed. The insulin didn't reduce my blood sugar much and the diabetes nurse said, "You're quite resistant to insulin." They advise against trying to conceive until my blood sugar is close to "normal." I've struggled with this sense that I am not doing well enough.

Lately, I have broken the cycle of guilt a bit by measuring my blood sugar two hours after every meal or snack, to try to observe in a less value-laden manner. I have discovered that rice paper rolls send my blood sugar up, as does oatmeal. Both are what I always considered "healthy" choices, but I've had to change the way I think about "healthy"—as "healthy" means different things to different people. I'm going to try a half portion of oatmeal cooked with full-cream milk, as I read a diabetes blogger, Chris Serong, say that he adds cream to his oats, because his body deals with the carbohydrates better when there is fat in the meal.[5] This is an interesting point because the message given to diabetics, and to people who are trying to avoid getting diabetes, is to "eat a low-fat diet." Yet I have also found that coupling protein and fat with carbohydrates gives me a lower blood sugar reading. In other words, melted cheese on a potato is better for me than just the plain potato. Yet low-fat recommendations are made, probably with the main goal being weight loss. However, if my main goal is lower blood sugar, and that is the road to "health" for me, that may conflict with guidelines for weight loss. I don't know why that surprised me when weight loss goals have been interfering with my physical and mental health all my life. The difficulty becomes when medical professionals advise you based on weight loss goals and you know that those goals aren't good for you; it sets up a situation where you don't know when you can trust the doctor. Questions like, "Are they telling me to do that because it might make me lose weight or because it's good for my health?" Or, "Do they have evidence backing up their advice, or is this based on old assumptions of what it means to be fat and have diabetes?" And, if I successfully become pregnant, when the time comes to advise on vaginal birth versus induction or cesarean birth, I will be faced with this again.[6] If they advise cesarean birth, my questions will be, "Do they think I'm not fit enough to give birth, because I'm fat?" and "They see being fat as a health risk, and being diabetic as a high risk; therefore are they always going to be overly cautious and protect themselves and recommend a c-section?" And the other question, "Are they right? Should I trust them? Maybe they are right—I can't tell. I'd better be cautious and trust them too." Which has led to me picturing and practicing with potential narratives that lead to cesarean section, to counteract the many years of assuming and hoping that I would have a natural birth. Accepting that by nature I am anxious and cautious, however much I'd like to be relaxed and spontaneous, is a part of accepting that I will probably listen to the doctors. With that comes acceptance that I may feel like I am betraying fat activism by not standing up and defying a weight-focused medical profession. When it comes to my own body, diabetes, and the medical profession, I don't know who to trust.

My grandmother died in her early seventies of heart disease—likely a complication of her diabetes. Yet she was never given medication to manage her diabetes, and I recently learned that, just as guidelines for body mass index and obesity changed to make millions of people obese overnight, artificially creating an obesity epidemic, so have guidelines for what makes a diabetic changed. In fact, my mum told me that when my grandmother was diagnosed, when I was a child, the HBA1C that made you a diabetic was considered 10 and over. That is considered incredibly high now, and my endocrinologist wants me below 6.5; and while I think that is a good thing, as it means fewer long-term effects of diabetes, it also means yet another "false" epidemic—the diabetes epidemic. Or that supposedly scary made-up phrase, "the diabesity epidemic." If diabetes thresholds were what they are today, all my diabetic relatives would have been early-onset type 2 diabetics, probably diagnosed in their thirties or forties.[7]

A year ago my mum started talking about joining the gym to help her knee replacement therapy. I had heard of a gym close to me that was run out of the

Royal Melbourne Hospital, with "no mirrors and no heroes." She wanted to go with me, for her rehab and to "support me." I went, and sometime after the eight-month mark I was sent a congratulatory letter saying "you've come to the gym 50 times since you joined." It averaged out to three times a fortnight, and that had been a struggle. There was rarely a day when I wanted to go. I went because forcing myself to do physical activity that I didn't really enjoy, that was repetitive and boring, was better than the fear I felt about my diabetes diagnosis—it was better than the guilt I felt when I didn't go. That should have been a wake-up call to me that something was wrong with forcing myself to go to the gym. Eventually, it was.

Sometimes when I went to the gym I was exhausted; often I was depressed; some days I didn't want to see my mother (who still has a strong weight focus), but I went. When I started to pull back and tell Mum I didn't want to go on a particular day, she would express disappointment; sometimes she'd say, "What's the point of me going if you're not going?" It became guilt inducing; so then I told her that, and she stopped doing it. But as I got closer to making a new year's resolution, I realized I didn't have the mental energy to force myself to do things I didn't want to do anymore—in general. Some switch flicked and I thought, it's not just the gym, it's everything—I don't want to be in that friendship, I don't want to go to the gym, I don't want to avoid that difficult conversation anymore—it was about facing up to how things are, accepting how things are, whether they were great or not. And not struggling internally with the conflict between who I am and who I thought I should be. That's around the time I told my dad I have diabetes, after delaying for almost a year. Mum said she was thinking of quitting the gym because it was expensive on her retirement wage, and I agreed that I wanted to quit too. It was a huge relief. My father didn't comment at all, and no one else really seemed to care that I didn't go to the gym anymore. I have mainly been walking my dog daily and doing some yoga off a DVD in the lounge room, and I kept thinking "I should do more," but these days I catch the "shoulds" and realize I'm doing what I'm doing, what I like to do, and that's what I'm going to do. In my life, it's been a challenge to actually do what I want to do, not do things I think I *should* do or that other people want me to do to please them or meet their needs. I marvel at those selfish types who seem to float through life with barely a consideration for other people, thinking only of their own needs, and possibly pairing up with people who do things they think they should do, rather than things they want to do. That's not what I want to (or could) become, but there has to be a happy medium. For me, this does link to my fatness, because the dieting was always about trying to present a particular image—being what society approved of—thin (or not big and fat, at least). The self-hatred of my body developed because society hates fat bodies, and my parents hate fat bodies. Using a barometer outside the self to judge the self is damaging when you're fat. And when I felt my body wasn't good enough, I also felt that I wasn't good enough.

Turns out the separation of the body and mind didn't work that well for me. This also links back to my career as an academic. I'm not going to generalize about all women, but I'm going to talk about my experience as a woman. I feel that society and the media continue to send women messages—that we are valued for our beauty first and foremost, that we should keep the peace and keep people around us happy, that we don't say "no," that our boundaries should be fluid, that showing strength, directness, and disagreeing with people is unattractive and unacceptable from women. I was told by my father, "You can have any job you want, you can be whatever you want," and I was also told continually, "You need to lose weight." So while he praised and valued me for my academic pursuits, he critiqued me for my "beauty," or lack thereof in his eyes. I remember thinking, just last year, "My father thinks I'm ugly," and I was a 35-year-old woman crying into my cup of tea because I think my father thinks I'm ugly. What does every little girl want? To be thought of as a beautiful princess? To be fair, I had fantasies of world domination, and at six years old I wanted to be "president of the world" and fix world hunger and poverty. I never wanted to be a princess, but I did still want to be a beautiful world leader.

Where does this fit with academia? I became an academic through my creative writing. I was studying journalism and creative writing and when I had to choose which to specialize in, I chose creative writing. My lecturer had told me to "watch the sunset" and "let it come to you." In essence, she was advising me to figure out what I wanted and who I was, not to do what I thought I should do. I instinctively chose creative writing. I'm not sure of the exact reasons, but I know that part of it was that as a journalist, I would be forced to write what other people told me to write about. Underlying my decision to be a creative writer despite the risks and insecurity attached to that (and not just "do" creative writing on the side) was a desire for change, yes a desire for people not to starve, which was my childlike view of how to fix the world, and that view of how to fix the world became more about accepting my limitations, and that there was no president of the world and even if there was one, I was unlikely to be it. And it became about new notions of what was wrong with my sphere of the world, and a lot of that was about revealing what goes on behind closed doors, what is considered taboo and "shouldn't be spoken about," about looking at what we accept to be true in the world, at the dysfunctional ways in which we manage to function as a society, and about how we judge other people's lives and choices, and also about the role of indoctrination—from school, work, medical institutions. About how hard it is to go against the grain and say "I'm not going to be what you expect me to be, or what I have been socialized to be," and when you've been socialized to be something that you then refuse to be, such as thin by dieting, or a woman who sets clear boundaries and sometimes says "no," you struggle with yourself as a socialized being, as well as the pressure and expectations from other sources.

Perhaps not everyone struggles with the self in such a way, but I do. Perhaps without my anxiety about the world, my place in the world, my ethics, my social justice beliefs, my queerness, my fatness—perhaps without my anxiety I would be without diabetes—I'll never know that for sure. But if anxiety is a contributing factor to diabetes, then it is also a contributing factor to being a creative writer, and a teacher and researcher, and I'm much more willing to take on "creative writer" as a label of who I am than "diabetic." I want to shake that "diabetic" label off and see it as something that does not define me. I don't want it to define me, but I have to take the label on board, if only to declare it, and in the same breath declare, I am human, I am complex, you don't know why I'm diabetic and you can't blame it on my fatness. Don't judge me, don't condemn me, don't scare me. Accept me, offer me assistance, trust me.

And with acceptance, acknowledge thatwe don't have complete control over our bodies or our health. It has felt like a burden I carry; I have felt less attractive because of it. No one can look at me and know I have diabetes, so when I question why I have felt less attractive, it is because I am labeled "not healthy," and sickness is seen as unattractive in our culture. Thin is equated with healthy in women, and muscular is equated with healthy in men, and anything outside those ideal body shapes is considered less healthy, and often less beautiful. I was able to turn my thinking around about fat—that I could be "healthy" and fat, which is one of the messages fat activists present— that you can't assume someone is unhealthy based on how they look. You can't know if a thin person is healthy. But to be diagnosed with type 2 diabetes at age 34, and to be bombarded with messages about lifestyle changes, weight loss, and health, is to feel unhealthy. My body is unhealthy. My body is fat. These two things don't need to be conflated to become "my body is fat and unhealthy" or "my body is unhealthy because it is fat" or "my body is unhealthy because of who I am and the choices I made"; but my mind is not a logical academic argument, so I have those thoughts, and I have become very self-protective and cautious and ready to go into battle with any new doctor I might have to see. I have become afraid of doctors' voices saying "you need to lose weight" or "you need to do better" or "you need to try harder" or "because you are fat you have diabetes."

I began to realize that the reason these voices, these statements, have the power to stab me is because these are thoughts, or subthoughts, I have been having. When I don't say them out loud, I try to pretend they're not there, and that has been a mistake. When the doctor says them, they resonate— what I had hoped wasn't true is being said to me—and while those statements are unfair, or perfectionistic approaches, or negative, they join forces with my own hidden thoughts and that is where the danger lies. I have been feeling like I want to be stronger and more resilient, and to be able to face those doctors and say, "You are wrong and I don't have to listen to this and I no longer want to be treated by you"; but in order to be able to do that, I have had to face my own dark thoughts and fears and accept that they're there—most are untrue, some are partially true, and their existence also needs acceptance. Did my binge drinking in my twenties lead to diabetes? Possibly, partially. Was that my decision and my fault? It was my decision—I am responsible for not tackling my heavy drinking before I hit 30 years of age. Did growing up in a physically and emotionally abusive environment with undiagnosed severe anxiety and depression and a sleep disorder lead to diabetes? Possibly, partially. Was that my decision and my fault? No.

Did I seek treatment? Yes, over and over again. Am I better now? Sometimes. It's a work in progress. Did dieting and binge eating high-calorie foods, and the subsequent weight cycling lead to diabetes? Perhaps. Was that my decision and my fault? I remember restricted eating from the age of four, my mum put me on my first diet at the age of eight, and I began secret eating and binge eating soon after. At what age did the dieting and binge eating become my decision and my fault? In a world where weight loss is the main health goal, coupled with my high-achieving mentality, the continued dieting goals were understandable. At the time, I blamed myself for the bingeing— it was a weakness, a failure in me. It was that sense of failure that led me to the Swinburne University mindful moderate-eating group. Once I was there, I began to see that I was not a failure and that the bingeing was a product of the dieting. But I also began to realize that, while removing restricted eating also reduced the bingeing, my body decided to be fat—fat even without the binge eating. These questions about how I got diabetes are perhaps futile, as are the questions about why I am fat. All the women in my family either are fat or were fat before they took up lifelong dieting. Type 2 diabetes is found on both sides of my family—so, genetically, I may have inherited genes from both sides. I may have switched those genes on with my lifestyle, but when I look at my life, it is hard to see a way that I could exist as me and not have diabetes. If it was inevitable, is it easier to accept? Easier to forgive myself for? Easier to think of as something that I don't need to forgive myself for? Maybe. I don't know yet.

It is beginning to seem futile to try to absolve myself of blame in an effort to end the negative feelings I have about diabetes. In *Against Health*, Kathleen LeBesco argues: "The fat person who argues moral validity by saying that he can't help being fat and has good eating habits and takes plenty of regular exercise seeks deliverance. It is an understandable goal, but one based on truly fraught reasoning that allows healthism to flourish unchecked."[8]

In essence, have I been fighting against a culture where healthism is flourishing, where it is considered an individual moral imperative to be healthy? Have I been trying to prove to myself that I didn't cause myself to get diabetes, and that if I did enact behaviors that caused my fatness or my diabetes, I am not responsible for those behaviors? In other words, I have been trying to prove to myself and to doctors that I am not lazy, greedy, gluttonous, and undisciplined, and that I do try to be healthy. I think it is important to acknowledge that while that is not a useful mind-set for living life, perhaps it is somewhat inevitable when interacting with the medical profession, especially when you have a chronic condition that requires substantial interaction with a range of medical professionals.

Sometimes I've questioned the label of "fat activist." I'm a writer first, then an academic, and while I thought of giving up my "dream job" as an academic, I would never give up being a writer. Some labels we take on and are proud of—we want them, they're desirable, they hold societal pull, we get respect for them. Labels like "creative writer" and "academic." Others people throw at us, and we reject them, like "a stiff"—what they called me in high school. So boring I was a stiff—a dead body. Other labels we take on are stitched into our bodies, in a bloody wound that heals. We grow to love them but know that we won't usually get societal privilege for them. "Queer" or "bisexual" were my first ones of this nature. "Fat" is one. "Fat activist" is another. "Diabetes" is one that infects me and that I keep trying to reject, with wishing I didn't have it, with avoidance of the care that the condition requires—the opposite of acceptance.

My fat activism involves occasionally talking to the media,[9] writing academically and creatively about fat,[10] and taking part in and supporting fat community events.[11] It is also privately commenting on antifat articles online, on medical "obesity" guidelines, on Australian curriculum guidelines about health and physical education for primary school students, and writing letters of complaint after seeing an antifat medical professional. It is a combination of public and private acts. It is not performing using my body, it is not wearing spandex, and it is not posing nude for fat artists—I admire these acts and love witnessing these acts but these are not things I would do, fat or thin. I challenge myself to write without censorship, to write without worrying about my students reading my work and judging me, to write without worrying that I reveal too much, knowing that "too much" is relative. I reveal myself, and I have revealed myself here, and it is essentially an optimistic act, to trust the reader, that you will read my lines and not between them, because I'm not writing between the lines, in metaphor or with deliberately missing information. I have resisted going back through this writing and censoring sections that show who I am too clearly. I have considered fat and diabetic in the written equivalent of a Venn diagram and discussed some of the major overlapping aspects of my life. My life is a work in progress and my perspective on fat and diabetes is evolving, which makes this chapter a snapshot more than a sustained argument.

In the spirit of a revealing narrative, I started writing this chapter before attempting conception, and I finish it now in the second trimester of pregnancy. Any more than that is a story for another time.

NOTES

1. J. Eric Oliver, *Fat Politics: The Real Story Behind America's Obesity Epidemic* (New York: Oxford University Press, 2006).

2. Samantha Murray, *The "Fat" Female Body* (Houndmills, Basingstoke, UK: Palgrave Macmillan, 2008).

3. Esther Rothblum and Sondra Solovay, *The Fat Studies Reader* (New York: New York University Press, 2009).

4. Linda Bacon, *Health at Every Size* (Dallas, TX: BenBella Books, 2008).

5. Chris Serong, "Move and Be Free," accessed May 1, 2013, http://www.move andbefree.com/1/post/2011/05/fat-acceptance-diabetes-and-health.html.

6. Pamela Vireday, "Women of Size and Cesarean Sections," Our Bodies, Ourselves, accessed May 1, 2013, http://www.ourbodiesourselves.org/book/companion.asp?id=21&compID=125#note22.

7. The Center for Consumer Freedom, "Changing Standards for Diagnosis," An Epidemic of Obesity Myths, accessed August 1, 2013, http://www.obesitymyths.com/myth8.2.htm.

8. Kathleen LeBesco, "Fat Panic and the New Morality," in *Against Health*, Kindle ed., ed. Jonathan M. Metzl and Anna Kirkland (New York: New York University Press, 2010), 76–77.

9. "Fat Fighters," *Insight*, SBS television, accessed May 28, 2013, http://www.sbs.com.au/insight/episode/watchonline/544/Fat-Fighters.

10. Jennifer Lee, "A Big Fat Fight," *Overland* 207 (Winter 2012), accessed August 3, 2013, http://overland.org.au/previous-issues/issue-207/feature-jennifer-lee/.

11. Va Va BoomBah, "Fat Burlesque Melbourne," accessed August 3, 2013, http://www.vavaboombah.com/.

6

Plus-Size Exercise: Coping with Fat Fitness, Stigma, and Stereotypes at Every Level

Jeanette DePatie

My first experience in hiring a personal trainer was not a good one. It was many years ago, while I was still an undergraduate in college. I had gained a little weight and I was feeling panic. I felt like I needed to "do something about it" right that very moment. I remember that I saw the name of a trainer posted on the bulletin board of my local gym.

Of course, before I started I did absolutely no research whatsoever about personal trainers. I didn't ask any friends or family who they thought was the best candidate. I didn't interview multiple candidates to see who was a good match for me. I didn't even interview the guy I eventually hired. I just took the number off the bulletin board at my local gym and called the guy up. "You gotta help me," I said. "I'm fat."

Eventually, I asked his price. For a kid working her way through college, that trainer's fee was a lot of money. But as I said, I was in a full-blown fat panic and was willing to do anything to get that weight off. I called my parents and asked if they would help pay for it. To put this in perspective, this was one of only two times I ever asked my parents for extra money to help me through college. I knew that they had scrimped and saved to help me pay tuition and expenses. I knew that asking for money meant that there were some things that they might need to do without. But I was so alarmed over this weight gain that I asked anyway. And my parents, sharing fully in my fat panic, complied.

My new trainer treated me with contempt from the beginning. He didn't really do much of a diagnostic with me. He tested me by plunking me on the treadmill. He later admitted that he was doing what we in the fitness industry call a maximum-exertion test. This means a test where the subject is expected to drop out at some point because he or she can't do it anymore. I felt like I was going to die on that treadmill. The trainer hadn't told me that it was a maximum-exertion test because he "didn't want me to wimp out." He had jumped to the conclusion that because I was fat, I wouldn't try very hard. He later admitted that he was very surprised that I completed the whole 15 minutes at that high incline level and speed. Yup, I completed it all right. And then I went in the locker room and threw up. I could barely walk for two days after that, but by golly, I completed the task put before me.

This exchange characterized our work together over the following months. He would work me to the point that I would usually vomit in the locker room after our sessions and collapse on the sofa at home. The day after our workouts, I was so stiff and sore, I could barely move. I barely had enough energy to get through the day. But I still had a full course load at college. I still had to go to work nearly every day to help meet expenses. I was paying a lot of money for the privilege of being abused every week and I hated it. I didn't dare tell the trainer I was hurting or sick or exhausted because he made it very clear that I should be ashamed of my body and that he didn't want to hear any "excuses" when I was exhausted or sick or in pain.

And of course, I wasn't losing weight—although the personal trainer had promised me that if I kept up my workout regimen and ate reasonably well, I should lose a lot of weight. I did what he suggested, but I didn't lose a lot of weight. The trainer accused me of lying about my training regimen and eating habits. When I asked for additional advice, he suggested that I stop lying to myself and to him.

Needless to say, something had to give. I grew tired of being tired and sick and in pain. I was finding it increasingly difficult to keep up in school and at my job. I wasn't seeing the results I had been promised. So, I quit. And as is so often the case, I didn't just quit working out with him, I quit exercise altogether for several years.

Unfortunately, this story is all too typical for fat people who seek help from the fitness industry. We run into personal trainers and exercise instructors who have never been taught to check their personal biases at the door. In fact, outside of repeating the same blather about calories in and calories out and a few vague warnings about knee and ankle joints, many personal trainers and fitness instructors have received no training whatsoever in helping them deal with the plus-size exerciser.[1] We are dealing with personal trainers and exercise instructors who don't really understand the temporary nature of weight loss or the myriad components that go into body size. Many of them truly believe that if you just do a little exercise and don't eat too many cheeseburgers, you can be thin.

I can say that my own training as a fitness instructor has been somewhat checkered. Luckily, by time I started on my journey to become a fitness trainer, I had personally done a lot of research about body size and health. I began my journey already understanding just how unlikely permanent significant weight loss was for most of my clients.[2] I also understood that fitness was one of the very best things my clients could do for their health, regardless of whether or not they lost a single pound.[3] I understood that much of the research I had reviewed went against the grain of what was commonly thought about exercise. I knew that most people felt that everybody could be thin if they only ate well and exercised. I knew that the research does not bear this idea out. I knew my viewpoint would be controversial with some. So I went in personally prepared for the prejudice I would likely face as a plus-size instructor. Or so I thought.

My first group exercise certification (not American Council on Exercise) wasn't too bad. Although I was the only person in the room with a double-digit pants size, the instructors didn't feel any reason to single me out. I was even complimented on my cueing skills. However, the first time I tested for my personal trainer certification (also not American Council on Exercise) was another story altogether. To be fair, I need to say that the actual written course materials were fairly good. There wasn't a lot of fat-bashing stuff in there and the statistics were pretty accurate so far as they went. The materials were guilty of some sins of omission. The books didn't include statistics showing how unlikely permanent weight loss is for most participants. But the statistics that were included seemed pretty accurate. Unfortunately, the instructors for the two-day intensive, personal trainer certification program didn't feel compelled to stick to the printed materials. Once again, I was the only person in the room with a double-digit pants size (well unless you count "00" as a double-digit pants size). Over the course of our two days together, the instructors went way outside of the printed materials to bash fat people and praise the noble thin instructors for dedication to "fixing the fatties." At one point, the instructor went to the white board and drew a crude picture of a person with a "hole in the middle of her body." The instructor then said, "That's why fat people need to eat and eat so very much. It's because they have a hole in their lives—something that is broken or not working within them—that they stuff with food." I wish I could say that I had acted on my first impulse—to stand up and ask the instructor to help me find the hole in my tummy—because I sure as heck couldn't find it. I wanted to ask her what evidence she had for making this assertion. Had actual research been conducted outside of what Cousin Sue told her aunt Flo? I wanted to call her out on her purely stigmatizing fat bashing. But you know what? I had paid every last dollar I had to take that course. And I knew that at the end of the course I would need to take two tests. One was a written test—which I felt pretty good about. The other was a practical test judged solely by this fat-phobic instructor. This second test was extremely subjective and I simply couldn't afford to take the test again. So I kept my thoughts about the holeyness of my tummy to myself and just got through it. I passed with flying colors. But the moment I received that certification, I wrote a scathing review of the instructor and complained about her to her superiors. You probably won't be surprised to hear that I never got any response to my complaints. I have never given another dollar to that certification agency.

So why am I going on at such length about my early fitness experiences and what I experienced in training to become a fitness instructor? I am going on about all of this because getting involved in fitness is one of the best and most important things I have done in my life. More than anything else, it helped me along my journey to feeling good and feeling good about myself. But because of the fat stigma rampant in our industry, this journey toward fitness almost never happened for me. And I believe that countless others find their fitness journeys cut off before they have even begun because of fat stigma. I believe that as fitness instructors, coaches, and personal trainers we have a duty to our clients. We are charged to treat them with respect. We are expected to help and not harm. We are supposed to know what the heck it is we are doing. But I believe, all too often, when it comes to our larger clients, we are falling down on the job. And I feel we are failing these fat clients in a number of specific ways.

WE FAIL TO TREAT OUR CLIENTS WITH RESPECT

I have certainly experienced prejudice, disdain, and outright contempt from other trainers I have met. And that's not really so surprising, because as far as the traditional fitness industry is concerned, a fat fitness instructor is an oxymoron.

In the traditional fitness world, teachers and gurus have the body that all aspire to. With a deep airbrushed tan and midriff bared to prominently display a perfect six-pack, fitness teachers are supposed to look like magazine cover models. Yoga teachers should look long and lean. Aerobics teachers should look lean with well-defined arm, leg, and abdominal muscles. Weight-lifting instructors should positively ripple with beefy biceps, huge quads, and prominent pectoral, deltoid, trapezius, and rhomboid muscles. And again, the glistening six-pack goes without saying.

As fitness teachers we are taught that our bodies are our calling cards. We are told that others will choose to work with us because they aspire to look "just like us." But there are a number of serious problems with this idea. One problem is that not all of us are even capable of looking like those magazine cover models—at least not on a long-term basis. Genetics play a strong role in our abilities to build and retain muscles. Many of us are not even genetically capable of developing a visible "six-pack." And what few people realize is that fitness modeling and professional competitive bodybuilding are often not at all about health. In fact both fitness modeling and bodybuilding are known to incorporate some rather dubious practices to get that "cut look" that is so desired. Many professional bodybuilders fight desperately to maintain muscle mass during the starvation phase that comes right before a competition. Many bodybuilders also intentionally dehydrate[4] themselves[5] before competition to "maintain their cuts," and it is not uncommon to see medical professionals standing by with oxygen tanks backstage during these competitions. Yet we fitness professionals often try to convince our clients that these bodies are the picture of "health."

Is it any wonder that fear and desperation around having an acceptable body for teaching fitness can make us teachers just a little obsessive about the way our body looks and more than a little cranky? Is it surprising that we have a hard time keeping body image issues in perspective when we work in an industry intent on scrutinizing every line and curve? Is it any wonder that some of us are disrespectful toward students who have a less than perfect physique?

In my career, I have experienced a number of fitness instructors who feel it is perfectly okay to use shame as a tool to "motivate" their fat students to lose weight. Inspired by media examples like the television show *The Biggest Loser*, teachers believe that by shaming their fat students, they are helping them. The problem with the shame approach to motivation is that it just doesn't work.[6] A study regarding the television show *The Biggest Loser* finds that viewers are less likely to exercise after watching the show and have a more negative attitude toward exercise.[7] And study after study show that shaming people does not lead to increased exercise activities, increased fitness levels, or weight loss. In the long run, people who are shamed are more likely to engage in addictive and dangerous behaviors and less likely to engage in positive health-giving ones like exercise.[8]

WE FAIL TO PROPERLY EVALUATE THEM

As a fat exerciser, I constantly face people making assumptions about my fitness level, my fitness habits, and my health. When I'm in the gym doing a workout, it's not uncommon for a complete stranger to tell me, "Good for you! You'll lose that weight in no time." Or sometimes people assume I'm a beginner and offer help: "Are you new to working out? Can I help you figure out how to get started?" And when I enter a class for the first time, I am often greeted by a teacher just radiating her certainty that I will drop dead in her class from a coronary incident without asking me anything about my current fitness level or experience. Even though I have been teaching fitness for more than a decade, I'm branded a beginner because I'm fat.

It's so easy to make assumptions about our fat clients. We have been conditioned by the popular culture and the media to see fat people as lazy, undisciplined, and incapable. In some cases, like that of my personal trainer, it leads us to ask too much of our clients. Since we don't believe they will do what is required, we ask for a whole lot in the hopes that they will do a little. In other cases, it causes us to ask too little of our clients. We assume that the fat client has no athletic talent or is incapable of doing much of anything, so we don't give her or him much of anything to do. There is no way to properly diagnose a person's basic fitness level just by looking at him or her. Luckily, there's a very simple way to gain a correct understanding of the fitness level of any client—fat or skinny. All you have to do is a proper intake interview and possibly a few simple fitness tests. It's proven, it's recommended, and it works. Now we just have to do it.

WE FAIL TO HELP THEM BUILD APPROPRIATE EXPECTATIONS

There's no question that people yearn for instant gratification. And in a world where contestants on shows like *The Biggest Loser* demonstrate 5- and even 10-pound weight losses in a single week, instant gratification seems possible.

So what's wrong with that? Why not let people believe that a "perfect" body is attainable and accessible to them, as long as it spurs them to exercise more? Even if we know that it is extremely unlikely that they will ever look like a pro bodybuilder or a fitness cover model, don't the ends justify the means? If promising them an amazing body gets them to work hard at exercise, and we know exercise is good for them, what's the problem?

In my experience, the problem lies with managing expectations. When we teach our clients to expect a certain kind of results, and over time they fail to see those results, a number of troubling things start to happen. One thing that happens is students get discouraged and they quit.[9] The reason is pretty clear. I often use the analogy of trying to get a kid to clean his room. If you say to a kid, "Clean your room and I'll give you a brand-new iPod," chances are that kid will clean his room. In fact that kid will be *excited* to clean his room. But if upon cleaning his room, the child is told he just didn't try hard enough, so instead, you'll be giving him an educational video about manatees, he's going to be pretty frustrated. Sure, you might get him to clean his room a couple of times, by promising that if he does it well enough, *this time* he will *surely* get an iPod. But eventually, when it becomes clear that the MP3 player is not forthcoming, he's not going to be interested in cleaning his room. And he's not likely to trust you anymore.

I've seen it over and over again. People begin making fantastic strides in their fitness levels. Ranika's functional fitness is up and her resting heart rate is down. She feels better, is sleeping better, and is even having better sex. But because her body doesn't look the way she hoped, she gives up right in the middle of these efforts—frustrated by what she perceives as lack of progress. Juan has been taught that progress means that he will have a body that looks like a model or professional bodybuilder. This is the "iPod" he was promised. And even though his quality of life is continually and significantly improving, he was never taught to see those things as progress. Naturally, Juan doesn't believe he is progressing. Naturally, Ranika comes to believe that exercise simply "doesn't work" for her. And before you know it, Juan and Ranika have given up on exercise altogether. What is most alarming is that Juan and Ranika may not just give up on exercise for a few days, weeks, or even months. They may avoid exercise for decades.

WE FAIL TO PRESCRIBE A REASONABLE AMOUNT OF EXERCISE

Another extremely troubling thing that happens when we don't manage expectations properly with our clients is that they come to believe that "more is always better." If a little bit of exercise is good, an extreme amount of exercise is way better. We watch contestants on *The Biggest Loser* exercise for hours. The contestants on this show exercise until they are nauseous, vomiting, or even actually drop from exhaustion. This quick-start, super-intense, boot camp mentality is the new normal.

But I can tell you that the number one problem that I've seen during my decade as a fitness trainer is that beginning exercisers tend to go out too hard and too fast. Doing too much too soon leads to pain and injuries. When exercise is too challenging, students quit.[10] And nothing derails a beginning exerciser quite like a major injury.

Injuries can be especially problematic for fat exercisers. As I saw in my own case, I was reluctant to tell my trainer when I was in pain. Clearly, my personal trainer was disgusted by my weight and felt that it signaled weakness and laziness. I didn't feel like I could say, "Hey, that hurts." I couldn't add more fuel to the fire of his prejudice. And when fat people are injured, they are often told by their trainers, doctors, and physical therapists that their injuries are caused by their fat. These fitness and medical professionals probably won't offer any evidence or even sound reasoning why this should be so; they just simply declaim it as simple fact. I am currently working on the Resolved Project with the Association for Size Diversity and Health along with the Size Diversity Task Force. In this project, people of size are asked to share their stories about their experiences with health care. I have been astonished by the level of body shaming experienced by these individuals at the hands of nurses, doctors, and other health care providers. And I have been particularly dismayed by the number of medical professionals who demand that their patients lose weight *before* they receive any other treatment. Never mind that there is no method for long-term weight loss proven to actually work in the long term. Patients are told that they can't get other treatments until after they lose weight.

Our fat clients may already be feeling panic about their fitness levels and their weight and body size before they even come to us. But all too often, we feed that panic—making vague threats about their future health, expressing disgust over the way that their bodies look now, and pushing them too hard and too fast for their comfort or even safety.

WE FAIL TO PROMOTE EXERCISE AS PLEASURE RATHER THAN PUNISHMENT

So often we are so worried about health outcomes and body size and other important metrics that we neglect one of the very most important aspects of fitness—fun. If I had a dollar for every time I heard a fellow fitness trainer talking about needing to work off calories to atone for various sins, be it the piece of pizza she ate yesterday or the 0.5 pound he gained last week, I could retire for life. But if I've learned anything in the past decade of teaching, I've learned this: people won't keep exercising if it isn't fun. Into every exerciser's life comes that moment where he or she has to decide whether to exercise, stay in bed for an extra half hour of sleep, or stay home and watch the latest episode of *Game of Thrones*. If the exercise isn't fun, if it isn't something the client actually looks forward to, he or she will inevitably pick bed or TV.

WE TEACH OUR CLIENTS TO FAIL AT FITNESS

When we tell our students that with moderate efforts with exercise and nutrition they can and will look like movie stars, we teach them how to fail at fitness. When we teach them to be ashamed of their bodies, to distrust the very important signals they are receiving from their bodies about hunger and pain, we allow them to be injured and to fail at exercise. When we teach our clients to see exercise as a punishment that they must endure as long as necessary to achieve an acceptable body size, we teach them another way to fail at fitness. We set them up to fail at fitness and then we blame them for that failure. But there is another way. There is a simple, effective, and proven method we can use to teach students of all sizes to enjoy a lifetime of successful and joyful physical movement. That method is called Health at Every Size or HAES.

THE HEALTH AT EVERY SIZE APPROACH TO FITNESS

Fortunately, there is an approach that is safe and effective and fun and proven to work. This is called the Health at Every Size or HAES approach to fitness and wellness. The Association for Size Diversity and Health offers the following HAES principles on its website:

1. Accepting and respecting the diversity of body shapes and sizes
2. Recognizing that health and well-being are multidimensional and that they include physical, social, spiritual, occupational, emotional, and intellectual aspects
3. Promoting all aspects of health and well-being for people of all sizes
4. Promoting eating in a manner that balances individual nutritional needs, hunger, satiety, appetite, and pleasure
5. Promoting individually appropriate, enjoyable, life-enhancing physical activity, rather than exercise that is focused on a goal of weight loss

Simply put, the HAES approach to fitness is about respecting and listening to your body, understanding that fitness is just one aspect of building a healthy life, and realizing that feeling good and experiencing joy are also important aspects of health. I have applied the HAES principles to both my fitness teaching and my own fitness practice over the past 10 years, and frankly, I have been astonished by the results. I have seen clients who could barely walk from the car to the classroom gradually improve to the point where they can exercise for an hour at a time, three days per week. I have seen diabetic students improve their blood glucose levels to the point that they could reduce their need for insulin injections or even eliminate the need for insulin injections or diabetes medications altogether. I have seen students suffering from depression build new social connections, get out of the house more frequently, and build happier and more rewarding lives. I have seen women who haven't gone dancing, worn a bathing suit, or gone out in public in years begin to do all of those things. I have seen clients who could once barely walk progress to the point where they can take the grandchildren to Disneyland for the entire day. I have seen myself progress from walking just a mile or two to completing a half marathon, triathlon, and full marathon.

Over the past 10 years, I have seen the benefits of the HAES approach and have applied it to my teaching in many important ways.

I LEARNED TO LOVE MY OWN BODY

As a teacher, I can say one of the most important things I ever did to help my students is to learn to love my own body—as is—warts and all. When I rejected the need to have a perfect, "postcard" body as a prerequisite of teaching, I removed a lot of pressure from my life. I was far less fearful, frustrated, panic-ridden, and cranky. Loving my own body makes it far easier to approach other people's bodies without disdain or disapproval. And by loving my own body, I present a better role model for my students.

I have also learned to reject the role of "poster child" for the size acceptance or size diversity movements. As a plus-size exerciser, I have experienced moments where people have put me on a pedestal as an example of a "good fatty" and set me up in opposition to a "bad fatty" who doesn't exercise. This is problematic for a number of reasons. First of all, there is no such thing as a "good fatty" or a "bad fatty." Second, being a poster child is too much pressure and too much work for anybody to have to live with. For years I was afraid to write my book and to speak out about size diversity because I thought I had to accept the role of poster child. "But what if I get sick?" I wondered. "Will I damage the movement?" Eventually, I came to understand that even with my moniker as The Fat Chick, I am *not* a persona, but rather a person. I am not an example or a paragon. I'm just a person. And since all people are imperfect, it is okay for me to be imperfect as well.

I LEARNED TO REDEFINE HOW FITNESS LOOKS

Almost everybody who has ever seen or heard the title of my book, *The Fat Chick Works Out!*, asks me the same thing, "Why do you call yourself that? Why do you call yourself The Fat Chick?" And I usually answer the same thing. I tell them that by calling out the fact that I am a fitness instructor *and* that I am fat, I am helping people widen their understanding of fitness. Some people who are fit look like magazine cover models. Some people who are fit look like Jeanette DePatie, aka The Fat Chick. Fitness looks different on every body. You simply cannot tell whether or not a person is happy, healthy, or fit just by looking at him or her. But there's room for every BODY under the fitness tent. You can declare yourself a successful exerciser even if you don't look like a model, even if you haven't lost a single pound, even if you are still fat.

I LEARNED TO THINK LESS ABOUT HOW BODIES LOOK AND MORE ABOUT WHAT BODIES CAN DO

When I learned to leave behind the notion that fitness has to look a certain way, I was free to start thinking about what fitness is. I learned to think more about what the body can do. And the more I thought about what bodies can do, the more amazed I became. Our bodies are magnificent! We can walk and skip and dance and swim and jump—practically without thinking about it. Were you to calculate the physics of catching a ball that somebody throws at you—to calculate the trajectories and compute the airspeed and the thrust against gravity—the math would be terrifying. Yet our bodies do these calculations instantly and constantly all day long. Throughout my own fitness practice, even when I didn't lose any weight, I *could* continually see progress in terms of what my body could do. When I trained for a half marathon, for a sprint triathlon, and ultimately for a marathon, I didn't lose a single pound. Had I calculated my success based on my weight, I would have seen the entire endeavor as a profound failure. In fact, had I been focused on the numbers on the scale, I doubt very strongly I ever would have completed any of those races. Seeing yourself as a failure week after week is not a winning strategy. But instead I was focused on what my body could do. Every month, my body could go farther and faster than it ever could before. I felt successful and strong and powerful. It propelled my training week after week. It propelled me 26.2 miles to the finish line. I have seen this excitement in my students year after year. I have watched them complete their first 10-minute workout and cheered with them the first time they walked a mile or the first time they swam a lap of the pool without stopping. I have laughed with them and cried with them and shared in their triumphs. It's wonderful and transformative and absolutely addictive. Celebrating the amazing things our bodies can do has kept both me and my students exercising year after year.

I LEARNED TO START FROM THE BEGINNING

The HAES approach suggests that we engage in physical activities that are "individually appropriate." We ignore this advice at our own peril. Over the years, I tried many times to leap out of the gate and begin my fitness efforts far beyond my fitness level. And each and every time I have done this, I wound up frustrated, exhausted, in pain, and injured. Then, after a few days, weeks, or months of being frustrated, tired, and hurt, I quit. Every single time, I quit. I never learned to succeed at fitness until I learned to begin at the level my body was at that very moment. This is also how I work with my students. I don't judge them based on where I guess they might be or where I think they should be. I simply meet my students where they are. If that means that the walk from the car to the class is all they can do that day, that's cool. That's their starting workout. I congratulate them for completing their workout and we celebrate their success. These students have already learned how to fail at fitness. I want to teach them to succeed. So I make sure they can and do succeed every single time we work together. And then we celebrate that success together.

I LEARNED THE IMPORTANCE OF CREATING A SAFE ENVIRONMENT

The HAES approach is about not only physical wellness but also social, mental, and spiritual wellness. If we want to help people with overall wellness, we need to create a safe place for them to work out. This means we need to create a space where others won't taunt, tease, or disparage them. This is why I don't say anything negative about my body in my classes. And this is why I don't allow my students to say bad things about their bodies or anybody else's body in my classes. If a student in one of my classes says she hates her thighs, I ask her to apologize to her thighs right there in class. I also ask her to publicly recognize and thank her thighs for all the wonderful things they do for her in her life. Calling out fat talk and fat shaming in a productive yet very public way helps drive home the need to be kind to ourselves and to our bodies. And feeling safe allows us to stretch and grow to our greatest potential. It also means that I confront bullies at the gym. If I hear about gym patrons making disparaging comments, or mooing sounds, or pointing, or laughing at, or teasing *any other gym patrons* for *any reason*, they hear from me directly.

I LEARNED TO HEAR MY BODY WHEN IT IS WHISPERING

The HAES approach is about being in tune with and learning to listen to your body. In the past, I had learned to ignore the signals from my body and to push through exhaustion and pain. The problem is that ignoring our body signals is much more likely to lead to burnout, dropout, and wipeout. That's why I've learned to hear what my body tells me while it is still at a whisper. When I pay attention to subtle aches and pains, I can learn to make small adjustments to my equipment (shoes, orthotics, clothes), my technique (stroke, gait, pace, position), and my program (duration, frequency, intensity) to improve my fitness experience. Small adjustments on the front end can save you from really big problems on the back end. If you don't listen to your body on the whisper, it will eventually yell and scream. And that is not good. I have also learned the importance of teaching my students to monitor what is happening in their own bodies. As a fitness trainer, it is my job to help them create and maintain the best program possible. But I am not privy to everything going on in their bodies. I can't watch every practice session and every bit of physical activity they do in their lives. So the more I can teach them to honor, interpret, and act on the messages from their own bodies, the better I can prepare them for a life of successful fitness.

I LEARNED TO SEE FITNESS AS JUST ONE PART OF LIFE

The HAES approach is about promoting all aspects of health to people of all sizes. That means that fitness efforts have to work as part of a whole life. Fitness efforts should be balanced with the need for rest, relationships, recreation, career, family, and all of the other responsibilities we face. When I worked with that personal trainer all those years ago, he failed to help me integrate fitness into the rest of my life. As a result, I quit. So when I work with my students, I try not to make hard-and-fast rules about what they can or should do. Generally, it's considered unsafe to increase exercise duration, frequency, or intensity by more than 10 percent per week. But that doesn't mean that students need to increase 10 percent every week. Students don't need to increase their fitness efforts at all, unless they desire it. And even when students make specific goals, like a 10 percent increase per month, those goals need to be flexible to accommodate real life. Is it final exams week? Are the kids home with the flu? Is your mother-in-law coming to stay for two weeks? Fitness goals may need to be adjusted. Fitness is not a short-term project. If it is going to be a lifelong process, it will ebb and flow. I find it helps to take the long view.

I LEARNED TO FOCUS ON FUN

The HAES approach specifies that exercise should be enjoyable. And if you want to stick to fitness for life, then you've got to find your fun. I've often said exercise is like sex. If you're not having fun, you're not doing it right. But that doesn't mean you or your students will find their perfect match right out of the gate. Sometimes people try a lot of things before they find the right thing. Joy and fun are absolutely critical elements of a successful fitness program. When I teach my classes I pay a lot of attention to the music I use and the choreography. I mix it up. Maybe one day I'll bring in scarves for the Bollywood routine or hats and canes for the jazz numbers. And I've learned not to take it personally when a student just doesn't find what I do or the way I teach fun. My methods are not going to appeal to everybody. That's fine. We all need to find something that helps us get out of bed and do our exercise while we record *Game of Thrones* on the DVR.

IN CONCLUSION

I've seen the fitness world from many different angles. At times I have failed as an individual exerciser and as an instructor. I've learned, the hard way, about many things that don't work. I've also learned from my own experience as well as those of my many hundreds of students what *does* work. And without a doubt, the thing that has worked best, the thing that has led to lasting joy and fitness success in the vast majority of cases, is the HAES approach. Thankfully, this approach is neither difficult nor expensive. It's available to people of all ages, shapes, sizes, and abilities. It's available to every BODY. I invite the fitness professionals of the world to adopt these simple yet profoundly powerful techniques to find joyful, lifelong health, happiness, and fitness for themselves and for each and every person they encounter.

NOTES

1. N. Robertson and R. Vohora, "Fitness vs. Fatness: Implicit Bias towards Obesity among Fitness Professionals and Regular Exercisers," *Psychology of Sport and Exercise* 9 (2008): 547–57.

2. L. Bacon and L Aphramor, "Weight Science: Evaluating the Evidence for a Paradigm Shift," *Nutrition Journal* 10, no. 9 (2011), doi:10.1186/1475-2891-10-9.

3. S. N. Blair et al., "Changes in Physical Fitness and All-Cause Mortality: A Prospective Study of Healthy and Unhealthy Men," *Journal of the American Medical Association* 273, no. 14 (1995): 1093–98.

4. Dan Gwartney, "Diuretics and Muscle Definition (Holding Water)," *Muscular Development* (December 15, 2009), http://www.musculardevelopment.com/store/ 1880-diuretics-and-muscle-definition-holding-water.html#.UapLs-u_GZY.

5. Bryan Denham, "Masculinities in Hardcore Bodybuilding," *Men and Masculinities* 11, no. 2 (2008): 234–42.

6. L. Vartanian and J. Shaprow, "Effects of Weight Stigma on Exercise Motivation and Behavior: A Preliminary Investigation among College-Aged Females," *Journal of Health Psychology* 13, no. 1 (January 2008): 131–38.

7. T. R. Berry et al., "Effects of Biggest Loser Exercise Depictions on Exercise-Related Attitudes," *American Journal of Health Behavior* 37, no. 1 (January 2013): 96–103, doi: 10.5993/AJHB.37.1.11.

8. L. R. Vartanian and S. A. Novak, "Internalized Societal Attitudes Moderate the Impact of Weight Stigma on Avoidance of Exercise," *Obesity* 19, no. 4 (2011): 757–62, doi: 10.1038/oby.2010.234.

9. Richard Ryan et al., "Intrinsic Motivation and Exercise Adherence," *International Journal of Sport Psychology* 28 (1997): 339.

10. P. Sullivan, "Exercise Adherence," *ERIC Digest*, ED330676, publication date 1991-00-00, ERIC Clearinghouse on Teacher Education, Washington, DC.

7

Fat Athlete

Sabrina Wilson

I've always thought of myself as an active person and enjoyed moving my body. I usually found my source of physical activity in the gym—the recumbent bike was my thing! That eventually evolved into taking group classes. I dreaded the standard aerobics classes, which always reminded me of the 1980s—and not in the good way. So, I eagerly got into more dance-style classes. My favorite was Samba. I loved the fast-paced rhythms and I loved even more that my fat body could not only outdance many of the other participants (much to their bewilderment), but I loved the way I looked doing it. I could feel it making me emotionally stronger as I learned to move my body without shame and with wild abandonment (have you ever seen Samba dancers' legs?!). I definitely felt like a "body outlaw." In what I have now come to define as my "fitness ADHD," I eventually grew bored with Samba and moved on to practicing NIA and then Zumba, both of which I initially enjoyed greatly but, like with Samba, grew bored with the repetition. Memorizing the routines to the point you can perform them at home tends to do that to you. I remember sitting there, in my car, in the garage, dreading going to class. I knew I had to make a change but wasn't sure to what.

Group sports!!! That will keep me challenged and engaged, right? It's not monotonous and repetitive—you have to stay quick-minded, on your toes! Plus, group sports were definitely a new experience altogether. I threw shot put and discus in high school, but that's about as solitary as you can get in group sports. I was looking for an activity that involved a community of people. Not only would this keep me more engaged, but it would hopefully fulfill the void of social interaction that I suspect is a contributing factor to how bored I get with individual physical activities. Even in a class, you still often feel pretty alone. Now, what sport? Soccer? I've always wanted to try it (especially after being discouraged as a seven-year-old when my not-so-present father told me I couldn't because I was too fat). Maybe volleyball! I could have a very powerful serve! So, I entertained the local community-based social sports league. The ones where it's more about flirting and the beers afterward. Kind of like extended Greek life for people experiencing their quarter-life crisis. I'm not judging—I still wanted to be a part of it!

However, I recall my first (and only) interaction with an organizer of the sports teams. I had perused the website and noticed two things: very few people of color and no fat people. It was very important for me to find a community that I felt comfortable and welcomed in. Research took up HOURS of my time. I'm not the go-and-see type of person to start with. But combine it with the knowledge that most spaces that revolve around fitness and activity are notoriously antifat and unwelcoming to body diversity—I was caught in a vortex of wanting to know exactly how awful it could be before having to actually experience just how awful it was. And for me, I could deal with being the only fat, black girl—I have dealt with that most of my life. It's not ideal—and frankly, it's boring—but I could still have a riot. However, I was hoping to research and discover that the culture of this social sports club was that everyone was accepted and all body types were embraced and they would love to expand the diversity of their participants. My e-mail to the organizer was blunt, "I don't see any fat people on your web site. Are the teams and sports not welcoming?" I'll admit that I kind of set my question up purposefully to see how they would respond to the word "fat" and what they would translate that to mean. Her e-mail back, although I'm sure she thought it was polite and sweet, told me everything: "Everyone is welcome. I will say that most people are pretty athletic, so you may want to keep that in mind." I didn't ask anything about athleticism, did I? Seeing the writing on the wall, I moved on. Clearly, an organizer suggesting that fat people *could* join, but keeping up is unlikely because being large equates to being unathletic, is not the team sport experience I would be looking for. Got it. Next!

I was still excited about a team sport though. Then I read an article about a local all-women, full-tackle football team. I remembered that a friend of a friend used to play and then I saw her name in the article. Eureka! I contacted her right away, arranged a meeting with the team owners, and before I knew it—I was signed up to play!

My family thought I was crazy. My mom was genuinely upset out of worry for my safety (a feeling that never went away and was later validated when I broke my hand in my last season). Honestly, I thought I might be nuts too. Tackle football? Full-on smash-mouth? Right, okay. Here we go! But even in my hesitation, I was convinced this was the place for me. Based on my conversations with the two owners, who said that big bodies were appreciated on the team and serve great purpose (one of the owners was a player and fat), and the photos I had seen, this team offered an experience that I was looking for. The women were ethnically diverse and there were plenty of fatties. Plenty of fatties running, jumping, and doing their thing. Yes, yes, YES!!

It was pretty soon into my first season that I started to realize that my teammates and coaches didn't really think the same as I did about body size and athleticism. And it wasn't until my second season, after the haze of my new endeavor waned, that I really began to be affected by the antifat nature of our team culture and also began to speak out against it. Finally, it wasn't until the end of my third season, with a broken hand that kept me out of championship game to boot, that as much as I loved certain aspects of being on my football team, I knew it was time for me to move on because navigating a space that seemed void of body positivity was just too emotionally and mentally draining—much more draining than the physicality of the sport.

On a (funny) side note: I will also say that my first season was kind of a wash for me. I was learning the game, absorbing the team sport culture (i.e., being totally okay with, as an adult, being screamed at and demeaned by our [male] coaches—a hard pill for this feminist to swallow). I conveniently refer to it as my really long practice for the following two seasons. My sister coined a great phrase that summed up what I looked like when I took the field: "chasing butterflies." While it was my job, as an offensive lineman, to protect the ball runners from the defense, which meant going out and stopping them— driving away their bodies with the force of mine to block access to the ball carrier—I was finding my tread. Thus, during that process, I would agree, it looked like I was trying to catch some butterflies—hands grabbing the air and everything. I thought I was trying to block, really. But it didn't really look like I was trying to tackle and stop the defense at all—just trying to catch some precious little fluttering butterflies, or a really awkward Monster Mash-type dance. It was entertaining (for my sadistic sister anyway). Dreadful (and hilarious).

But at the same time as I was learning the sport and coming to understand how players and coaches thought and behaved, more importantly for me, my first season marked the period I was getting in shape—a level of fitness that I knew I desired for my body to perform best in my position and a level I had never achieved before. My aerobic endurance had tripled, at least. A season before, running a flight of stairs left me breathless for many seconds. After my first season and a full summer of intense training, I could take the three flights in my apartment building at almost full speed and barely have an increased heart rate. I was amazed. My agility had improved drastically as well. I could move and pivot my body with ease that would be incredibly useful on the field. I was also amazed at the strength I had built. Workout routines that included flipping and dragging tractor tires, multiple planks, and countless kettle bell thrusts left my body incredibly strong. When I got into my lineman stance, I could feel the power in my quadriceps and butt muscles, charged and cocked with the immense force needed to drive opponents out of the way. Above it all, however, I felt tremendously fit. Fully aware that as a society we use that word almost exclusively with thinness, I always rejected that, and even more now. Who could deny that my athletic prowess wasn't evidence of being fit? To put it in perspective, most people I knew (of all sizes) couldn't keep up with my athletic training, so it made sense to me that I could confidently identify as a "fit" person. However, even though I felt in great shape by season two, my self-understanding of fitness and athleticism was apparently delusional according to the groupthink mentality around athletic performance and mere body size. For my second season, the team was revitalized and under new ownership, and everyone was hyped up and eager to put the new team on the map. Now, I really felt like a football player. An athlete.

I was still so confident that full-tackle football would be an environment that embraced fat acceptance, as well as gender nonconformity and the resistance to conventional body ideals that go along with it. But this was only because I made several incorrect assumptions. Each of those assumptions was eventually challenged by the reality of the team experience.

First of all, it's all women playing full-tackle football. I naively thought the team had to be filled with like-minded feminists. Women proving they can do just as the men do against sexist societal expectations. Yet despite the revolutionary steps they were taking in the world of football, the actual culture I experienced seemed entirely void of any sense of feminist or queer politic and totally acritical about the significance of having all female players and all male coaches. Perhaps it was because so many players had been lifelong athletes (basketball, softball, soccer) that being a jock was first nature, having male coaches was the norm, and the fact that their new sport of choice was football didn't seem that socially progressive, even though it's almost the only major sport that women are systemically shut out of on a precollege, collegiate, and professional level. But for me, part of the allure of joining this sport was because of the sociopolitical statement I thought it made. It was a "fuck you" to the naysayers who proselytize on women's inability to physically compete at the level that male athletes do. It's a definite sense of pride and bravado to have been able to say to people that I played football. "Oh, you mean flag football?" Except for the fact that I'm fat, most men wanted to ask if it was the football league where the women dress in their underwear (the name that shall not be spoken!). "No, it's full gear, full tackle." I lived for those jaw drops. All of the players had similar stories and they too beamed with pride when people were in awe that they were women playing football. However, there was a contradiction in thoughts around gender and sports that existed. The pride in being female football players coincided with the fact that so many players wanted not to be recognized as women playing football, just players playing football. The general consensus seemed to be that we should publicly express ourselves as players first, women second. The only exception was that almost every press release I saw from our team or the league spoke about the phenomenon of us being women playing football, although the statements didn't offer any further political or social commentary. This always seemed a disservice to the contribution we were making to the sport. Something I still don't fully understand.

However, what seemed to me as the "gimme" as to why this sport and these teammates would embrace size diversity, specifically, was because so many players were actually fat. Gloriously fat! But it wasn't that I assumed that being part of an oppressed group immediately led to consciousness of that oppression. My assumption stemmed from the fact that they were fat and their size was used as amazing leverage to be the most powerful players—particularly for the linemen. I had the initial impression that this was celebrated. One of my favorite things was to watch two 300-pound women, in full gear, go at each other as they used the momentum of their body weight coupled with bulging muscle to grapple and see who could win a match of "King of the Hill." And it wasn't just me that reveled in this. So many players talked about the biggest players in, what I thought was, total admiration. "Holy shit, did you see her pancake that linebacker! That was fucking awesome!" These were fat bodies training and doing drills in practice, only to play victoriously against opponent after opponent. This was indeed something to celebrate and seemed a natural conclusion, and proof positive, that size could not be exclusive of fitness level. It required stamina, endurance, and power. It seemed the perfect recipe for everyone involved to appreciate fat bodies and see that being fat, after all, isn't synonymous with being lazy and unathletic.

Where was the disconnect? Why was I constantly faced with narrow visions of athleticism, incessant diet talk and fat hate speak, and the general dismissal of any sociopolitical significance that existed in the sport? Here are some defining moments that demonstrated the problems with my assumptions about playing football and how I thought it would be an affirming, positive experience. As I will discuss throughout the chapter, in retrospect this experience also gave a lot of insight into the challenges faced by women's team sports on the pathway to empowering female players.

"SHE'S ATHLETIC"

I was at practice and my offensive line coach was explaining a certain technique to me and stated that the "athletic players" were more successful with the movement. It wasn't the first time that he said something alarmingly sizeist. However, this time I challenged him on it. I told him that I understood he meant "thin" when he said "athletic" and that I found his comfort in the

interchangeability of those two words to be incredibly problematic—
especially for an offensive line coach. The offensive line is a group of players
who are usually expected to have substantial size and girth, combined with
immense muscle and agility, to create a huge force to be reckoned with on
the field. And these are athletes. Athletes who are athletic—in that their
training and strength ability serve a specific and meaningful purpose within
the sport. Some players are better, more seasoned, or naturally talented in skill
than others—but all are athletic as long as they're training and performing
their role in the game. So there I was, my coach telling me that I'm not athletic because my body didn't fit his prototype of athleticism, which in turn tells
me that almost none of my fellow lineman were athletes either, according to
his standard. When I challenged Coach's comment, he did become defensive,
not combatively so, but stumbled around to say that, yes, the fat linewomen
were technically athletes, but that the thinner players offered something that
I couldn't achieve. Granted, I think that this person seemed to usually be
quite frazzled by my ability to intelligently converse with him. It could be
because he was 20-plus years my senior, or because he was a white man that
didn't expect being challenged by a black woman, or because I never really
got accustomed to the whole "Do as I say and say it with 'Yes, sir' " culture that
seems to be a huge part of the player-coach dynamic within team sports. So it
was not uncommon for my questions to be dismissed and this time was no
exception. Without skipping a beat, he continued to refer to thinner players
as athletic. I continued to be infuriated and discouraged by the knowledge
that not even my own coach considered me a true athlete because I was fat,
and at the very least he was never interested in understanding that many of
the ways he spoke would never communicate that he thought we were
athletes.

"TO THE FENCE AND BACK"

I am a firm believer that there is no one definition of a "fit" body or what an
athlete looks like and that different bodies can bring different skills. So, what a
fit offensive guard looks like and has the ability to do is likely quite different
from what a fit running back looks like and has the ability to do. This idea
was most relevant to some of the conditioning exercises we did. There was a
lot of running—A LOT! Now, I know there are fat folk who are great long-
distance runners and just enjoy running in general. However, the big bodies
on a football team are not (typically) marathoners in training. We were all
about short bursts of speed and massive power—often not moving more than
15 yards. But every practice started with what seemed like endless running.
Penalties earned in the game equaled punishment dealt in 100-yard sprints—
multiple times. In a row! If we were slacking off on the sidelines or during

conditioning, the coach would yell, "To the fence and back!!!" I dreaded those words—makes me shudder, still. This meant a sprint totaling about 250 yards, then back to conditioning. And if we didn't make it as a group— as in the slowest of us keep up with the fastest—we did it all over again. I recall running to the fence and back for more than a half hour straight. The players who excelled in running on the team would initially run so far ahead that we were screaming for them to slow down. Then, one or two charitable souls would turn back (I don't think they were even breathing hard) to run along-side the slowest of us (I was usually one of them) to encourage us to the finish line. That was very nice of them, but I tried not to look up and see the utter rage on the faces of the faster players waiting at the end. Their voices yelled, "Come on, Wilson! You can do it!" But their faces screamed, "Come on you out-of-shape fat ass! You're going to make us run again if you don't hurry up!"

The linemen of the team weren't lazy at all. We just couldn't run as fast as the smaller players, especially for long distances. So as a method to make con-ditioning make more sense for us, several of the linemen got together and peti-tioned to have drills built just for us. Still tons of running. But the distances were short and more meaningful to the type of power and endurance I wanted to build. The reaction of the smaller players was often that we were being lazy and it wasn't fair. Or, if they weren't totally negative about it, it was clearly out of expressed pity because we were unable to keep up. I admittedly despise run-ning and confess that I may have been especially embittered toward how much of it there was. Perhaps it is normal for collegiate or pro football teams to require everyone to run as much as we were. So for players where their life is supported by their athletic performance (paid or academically), maybe the expectation that all players run at the same level is reasonable. But for a semi-pro, community-based football team, I thought that expectation was out of focus. Therefore a solution of equal time running, but a different structure of running, seemed like a great compromise designed to improve team perfor-mance within the limited time available to volunteer players.

I recall one of our talented wide receivers lamenting on this "unfairness." I asked her, "Do you think it's possible that different bodies excel at different activities?" I went on to explain that from my point of view, running long dis-tances, although still a form of aerobic conditioning, didn't make sense to me if the expectation was that it was preparing us for the game. I've never seen a lineman run long distances over and over again on each play. So if the goal was to increase our endurance and athletic conditioning, perhaps a better method would be drills, including forms of running, that translate to the field for us. Sprints in short distances of 5–30 yards, multiple times, made sense to me. I run like that in a game, and running these drills repeatedly in practice would absolutely build my endurance. More importantly, I continued to explain to her, was that besides my own admitted hate of running, why is it that one activity, at one specific standard of performance, is used to judge athleticism or endurance? There is no way I can run as fast as a running back—even on a jog—and keep up that pace for 100+ yards. That doesn't physiologically make sense. Finally, I drew a comparison for my teammate to fully illustrate my point. "If you think the drills linemen do are unfair to everyone else, how about you really level the playing field? For the next drill, you can drive a 300-pound player back 10 yards, succeed, and then do it again about 10 times, at the same level that us linemen do it." I added that it was important that it be a lineman opponent as well, because the running required was at the level of players who sprint up to 75 yards multiple times throughout the game. She was quiet for a few moments and then responded, "That's a really good point. I've never thought about it that way." I had this exact conversation about two other times during my tenure on the team. Unlike this one exchange, the typical response was incredibly dismissive, often from other fat players who just seemed to hate their own fat body that, ironically, served them such great purpose in their team roles. Eventually, the linemen-specific drills were eliminated (due to too much objection from other players) and we were back to running with the runners, and being yelled at for being out of shape and lazy.

"BBU"

My disillusionment in thinking that football would be a body-positive experience took the sharpest turn at the beginning of my third season. At the beginning of the season prior, I actually felt really good. There was some of the usual sizeism talk, but the camaraderie and positivity among the bigger players seemed greater and genuine. I had formed a particular trust with one player who I even worked with to petition the linemen-specific drills that I described in the previous section of this chapter. We would often joke, even with self-deprecating humor, about being fat. But I was comfortable with it. I had no reason to think it came from a place of self-hate or size bigotry. It certainly didn't for me.

One of the ongoing jokes, born out of our petition, was that we were now "Big Bitches United"—the "BBU." I thought it was silly and cute—but affirming and proud. Mostly, I just didn't take it very seriously. But as the season went on, things started to shift. There were new groups formed that designated other "supportive" subgroups, like less-fat women and another group of BBU allies who defined their allied role because they were thin but liked to eat a lot. It was the fat girl in a skinny girl's body trope. I'm thinking, "Oh, please stop this train, I need to get off now." And it just digressed from there into much worse territory.

The conversations surrounded wanting to move from one group to another, by dieting, with "BBU" seeming much more of a derision than anything else.

I eventually removed myself from the ongoing joking, and if anyone referred to me as BBU, I quickly demanded that I not be included. Of course this began the "Sabrina and her weird pro-fat stuff" looks (pretty much just rolling their eyes with an exacerbated sigh). True, I might have been a bit of a killjoy for what most thought was a pleasant, playful joke. However, not only was I offended that "BBU" had become a "laughing-at-you" kind of joke, but I was utterly perplexed, and incredibly disappointed, that this new form of all-too-familiar diet talk was so embraced by this specific group of women. Women who through their athleticism, queerness, ethnicities, sizes, and/or gender expressions were totally atypical to conventional forms of femininity and socially subscribed gender roles. One minute they're comparing each other's fat rolls and detailing how disgusting they are; the next moment they're hurling their body and brute strength to sack the QB. How could we be in a place where we are defying the myths about the lack of female power and athleticism to play the hypermasculinized, historically sexist sport of football, but have no critical theory to bring to the table when it came to shaming our bodies and idolizing only one vision of a "good body"?

By the end of the second season, I felt deflated. But the third season was much worse and was the beginning of the end of my participation. The very teammate that started "BBU" as a positive statement of empowerment (or so I thought) underwent weight loss surgery. She returned much, much smaller to the welcoming hurrahs and congratulatory sentiments on her changed frame. I should add that prior to her surgery when she announced her plan to me (on my Facebook wall of all places), I made my opinion known that I think weight loss surgery is always a mistake. So when the BBU jokes immediately started again, and she knew I hated the joke and we weren't really on speaking terms, the entire conversation took a much more vindictive turn. One day she announced that apparently BBU didn't describe the fat women on the team well enough. "All them girls who are more than 300 pounds, they're 'Moo Cow.'" The laughing roars of "Dang, that's harsh!" and "You're so cold" were in jest—not objection. She justified it by saying that she used to be "Moo Cow" and it was disgusting. I stood nearby, gearing up for practice, with no choice but to overhear this very loud proclamation of absurdity. Mostly, I thought to myself that I couldn't believe this was an actual conversation *among football players*. This stereotypical mean-girl mentality and behavior that women use to denigrate other women based solely on body size and weight was being performed in full gear, on a field, about to smash bodies. Not to mention she was still a lineman, and many of the women who were her fellow linemen were, in fact, this disgusting group of "Moo Cows," including me.

This team, which I had hoped to find some body-accepting solace in, was little more than a replica of what I encounter every day—offensive, unfounded bigotry driven by pitiful self-hate and unreasoned beliefs about what fat bodies are and can do. It was a perplexing and frustrating paradox of women who represent the antithesis of societal status quo of what women should be, in terms of gender expression, femininity, and athletic ability, but at the same time being a group of women who were quick to embrace and depend on the toxicity of body hate and thinness adulation.

As I ended my third season knowing I would not be returning, I thought to myself: why does the body shaming exist? Perhaps it was because that even though everything about my experience screamed atypical—full tackle, primarily queer-identified women of color—this same group of people, despite all of this, are so ingrained with socialized antifat messaging that there is no escape. The challenging of the status quo stopped at the ability to think about the very definition of "athlete" in a more critical way. I wonder if it is because there is a point where marginalized groups of people (women of color, queer, female athletes) simply can't add one more identity or status (fat) that they have to fight for—politically or personally. Further, my limited experiences with teams in the other cities we played did not suggest that this phenomenon was specific to the city I was in. I still hold hope that those involved in the sport will evolve to think of themselves as the perfect group to challenge the definition of athlete as only a thin person, the same way they have challenged the definition of an athlete as only male, and to champion the power that women *and* diverse bodies bring to the sport.

Undoubtedly, I don't think my entire experience in football was awful. I made friends who inspire me and who I still hang out with today. But more so, it was an amazing test of my physical ability and really challenged my emotional and mental capacity for dealing with fat hate and thriving despite it. I chose to go back to every practice and, in my strongest moments, publicly confronted those who spoke with voices of sizeism. I don't think I changed the minds of most of the people I have met and interacted with during the three seasons I played, but I do think some took pause at what they were saying. For a moment, our fat-bodied contribution wasn't invalidated, and I found that meaningful.

Playing football also challenged my own thoughts on healthism. When I started, I thought this was a surefire way to be a "good" fat person. One who was active and working to be fit. However, still being incessantly judged as less than made me rethink that bias. After all, regardless of my physical activity level, it appeared that I would never be thought of as an athlete, and certainly not healthy nor fit. This is absurd. Not just because I was certainly an athlete or because it's untrue that fat people can't be fit and healthy, but mostly because that's not the point. The opportunity to feel dignity and self-respect shouldn't be solely derived from exhibiting "good" or "healthy" behaviors. Whereas I experience joy and fulfillment in physical activity,

I have plenty of different-bodied friends and family who do not enjoy it and have no interest in it. And who cares? Even if I agree that physical activity can potentially provide health benefits, it is not a guarantee; but even if it was, it's not anyone's business to declare someone morally obligated to do so. Health status or athleticism cannot be a factor in determining human worth.

Ultimately, being a fat woman while playing for my former team has also allowed me to grow in how I deal with fat hate in the outside world. Playing a team sport is not just like a second job; it is this microcosm of community—one that I thought would be very different from the external world but turned out to be quite similar in its stigmatization of fatness and rejection of body diversity. But that microcosm of a community tends to make experiences that much more vivid and in your face. There seemed no escape from it most of the time. It's a challenge, unlike what I've experienced in the "real world," to maintain my sense of self-confidence and body pride when, even while you are accomplishing great feats along with these family members, you are still told that your body is wrong. Somehow, the intimacy of that body-hating experience has given me space to feel more courageous about addressing bigotry even when out of the pads and off the field.

Today, I still find myself in football recovery—the addictive nature of the adrenaline rush from playing a team sport—as I continue to search for an activity that gives me the same thrill. But I am also searching for the cathartic space to heal from the emotional stress I experienced while participating in football, and I am more focused in finding, or creating, an experience where my own body positivity will be embraced and nourished.

8

Fat Athleticism and the Impolitic Body

Jayne Williams

I did not expect the meat pies to be so large. They bulged and glistened in the metal food service tray like turnovers on steroids. Some of the bigger ones were eight inches wide. The northwest Louisiana town of Natchitoches is best known as the setting of the chick flick classic *Steel Magnolias*. On the third Saturday of September, though, Natchitoches is the home of the World Meat Pie Festival, Meat Pie Eating Championship, and Meat Pie Triathlon, and I was a last-minute entrant in a competition that I hadn't originally signed up for. I stared at my tray of meat pies, wondering if this was a good way to spend the afternoon before a triathlon.

I confess: I knew full well that all the meat pies I could eat in a 10-minute period would not be the ideal prerace meal. I had already sampled a few of these, and while the succulent combination of meats, onions, and spices was delightful in a wrapping of deep-fried pastry dough, there was no way that multiple meat pies in one sitting was going to be anything but a gut buster.

My road to this tiny town, a literal backwater, was meandering. I had an idea that doing triathlons all over the country would help me sell my book about triathlon's many charms, and that maybe I could write another book about the traveling and the triathlons, and about all the enticing food I would eat on my travels. And what part of the country has better eats than Louisiana? Googling for "triathlons in Louisiana," I came across the Meat Pie Tri, and so my fate was sealed. I did not plan, however, to be standing on a stage, preparing to choke down meat pies at speed.

Ideally, on the day before a race, the serious triathlete would do a short workout in the morning, maybe a half hour on the bike followed by a 20-minute run, and then stay off her feet the rest of the day. Instead, I strolled the grounds of the Meat Pie Festival on the shores of the Cane River Lake. Was it a river? It looked like a river, except it didn't move. Was it a lake?

Turned out it was a lake that used to be a bend in the Red River, then the river changed course.

I was already feeling kind of drained by the time the World Meat Pie Eating Championship was getting ready to kick off. It was 95 degrees and Louisiana-humid, and I felt I should retire to the four-poster bed at my B & B for some air-conditioned prerace visualizing (aka napping). But then I saw Keri, the head contest honcho, who also happened to own that B & B, bringing huge trays of meat pies onto a stage. One guy, noticeably fatter and older than the beefy college kids who would be stuffing face to chase the glory and the $500 cash prize, turned out to be "Gentleman" Joe Manchetti, a professional competitive eater who has scarfed against the best in the world.

Keri grabbed a microphone and exhorted the crowd to step on up. "Let's get some women up here, come on!" I felt a twinge of competitive ego raising its head. I mean, I know from long experience that I can eat more than most gals, and a lot of guys too. But no, I shook my head. I was doing a triathlon tomorrow, for cryin' out loud. I went off and bought a lemonade and came back to the stage to watch. And suddenly I experienced an irresistible urge to eat competitively, in public. "Oh, what the heck," I proclaimed to Keri. "Sign me up." "Yay!" said Keri. Another woman also entered the fray, a petite Brazilian student named Erica. I figured I had the women's division sewn up.

I was nervous on stage. This was my first foray into competitive eating. Would I make a mess? Would I hurl in mid-bite? What would the crowd think of me, a demonstrably fat woman, getting up on stage to reaffirm their stereotypes about fat women? This was socially more risky than being a fat woman wobbling down the road in spandex and running shoes. At least jiggly jogging shows the uninformed observer a dedication to becoming less fat, whereas entering the meat pie-eating contest seemed to demonstrate dedication to the opposite.

The organizers counted out 8 meat pies per person, with the exception of Gentleman Joe, who got 17. I guess Keri wanted the record of 16 pies to fall. We each got two plastic cups of water, to help wash it down. I tried to establish camaraderie with Erica, but she had her game face on, or she didn't see the inherent weirdness in the event. She ignored my ingratiating grins and Groucho eyebrows. We were going to have 10 minutes to eat. Keri's volunteers placed plastic puke buckets behind us, which made me feel odd.

The announcer counted us down. I grabbed my first pie and took a big bite. Mmm, tasty. The first one went down fast; I grabbed the second. Took a little longer, but still tasted pretty good. On the third one, the dough started to seem glutinous. I looked around as I chewed. Gentleman Joe was well ahead, but everyone else seemed to have about the same size pile of pies as me. Erica was a full pie behind. Meat Pie Number Four didn't taste particularly appealing, and I started to think about walking away from the fray. Everyone was slowing down, but I grabbed Number Five.

By this time I was looking for pies with less dough on the edges, as crust was definitely the hardest to get down. The filling was easy to swallow without a lot of chewing. I sipped water as I went, trying to strike a balance between washing it down and further distending my stomach. The sixth meat pie just looked revolting. But my competitive fire was burning, and I figured I could give it a shot. I munched mechanically, trying not to taste. As the crowd counted down the last 10 seconds, I popped the last morsel in. I wasn't sure if they'd count the whole pie if I hadn't swallowed it all by the whistle, so I gritted my teeth and gulped.

We stood around holding our swollen bellies as the judge came by to certify our scores. First guy, 6½, a disqualification for puking, 10 pies for Gentleman Joe, 4 for Erica, 6 for Dave the college student, and so on. Most of the nonpro guys were somewhere between 5 and 6¾ pies, so my 6 put me squarely in the middle of the pack. Obviously, I kicked Erica's ass, but alas—competitive eating doesn't have men's and women's divisions. But even though I was not formally announced as the new women's World Champion Meat Pie Eater, I knew that's what I was. I did puke later that afternoon, intentionally, and not for the first time in my life.

The next morning, I did complete the Meat Pie Triathlon, though not quickly. I wasn't last, but I wasn't winning any prizes, even in the slightly fatter-athlete division. But that's where I often place, so I'm not sure if the pre-race meat pie extravaganza had particular deleterious effects. The Cane River Lake was warm and the color of iced tea, the neighborhoods across the lake were cypress laced and quiet as we ran through them, and I was not bitten by a snapping turtle during any portion of the event. Nobody said to me, "What's a fat cow like you doing in a triathlon?" Nor had anyone said, "What's a fat cow like you doing in a meat pie-eating contest?"

An interesting intersection of food, athletics, bulimic behavior, social mores, competitiveness, and psychology. I had ambivalence about engaging in competitive eating as a fat woman. On the one hand, I was reluctant to be seen as everyone's stereotype, the gluttonous overeater who probably eats like that all the time. But part of me wanted to say, hey, you know what? I can eat a bunch and I don't care who sees me do it! I want you to see me. You think I'm a fat pig? Fine and fuck you, I'm a fat pig. I'm gonna eat six meat pies and I'm gonna do a triathlon tomorrow. My body is big and fat and strong and now it's right up in your face. It is the Body Impolitic.

I was a "good eater" from earliest infancy. According to my family, the only thing I ever spat out was puree of beets. And who could blame me? (I have to mention, out of fear of reprisal from the Root Vegetable Anti-Defamation

League, that I like beets now too, though not pureed beets.) No cute little games were required to get me to eat, no "here comes the airplane into its hangar" or "how does the little froggie open her mouth?" Nope, not for me. I ate willingly, avidly, with evident enjoyment. Could I have been born with highly inclusive taste buds, preformed to savor the flavor and texture of just about everything?

I've been athletic and big and strong since I was a kid. Even before I fit most people's definition of "fat," I was tall and robust and round, not slender, definitely not girly. Though not the victim of merciless and constant taunts, there were enough playground slights and snickers that I knew I was the Chubby Girl. I'm fat now, it's true. My early start as a "good eater" put me on track, not very much later on, to be an early dieter.

I don't know if my attempts to lose weight early in life messed up my metabolism so that I later became fatter than my genes had originally suggested, or whether I was headed toward full-on fatness all along. As it was, it took me until my late forties, and many diets, and many years of eating to reach the 300-pound mark. I've looked at food in some sick ways, and I've eaten food in some sick ways as well as in some healthy ways. At times, I've tried to atone for calories in a joyless grind of exercise, and at other times I've eaten nourishing food and moved my body because it felt good to move it.

As a kid, I ate up sports and games. Red Rover? Hell, yeah, I'll come over! At home in the neighborhood, we hurtled around on primitive skateboards and built bike jumps out of scrap plywood, propping the rickety structure up higher and higher to get more air. That phase ended after I got too much air and landed squarely on my tailbone.

At school, we played an anarchic tackle football game with the distasteful name of "Smear the Queer," which involved everyone piling onto on whoever had the ball. I assumed a "queer" was a synonym for "it," as in "you're it." I kicked the kickball, dodged the dodgeball, and tried my hand at soccer and field hockey when P.E. threw those sports our way. I wasn't a gifted runner, though, especially the kind of continuous motion and sprinting required by soccer. I liked the kicking, but I tired pretty easily.

In fifth grade I added basketball and volleyball to my repertoire. I basked in my reliable coordination, my aggressiveness, and my strength. I always wanted to be tough; I never cried, never backed down. If I fell down, and I did, often, I got back up, brushing off the dirt and panting but ready to go again. I don't know where the drive to toughness came from. Maybe it was from reading old-fashioned children's stories of cowboys and the West, or of kids with brave dogs who solved mysteries and never whined. Maybe it was just some self-protection I decided was necessary at an early age. I just wanted to be a tough girl, one who never had to wear ankle socks with little frills. And I understood that toughness could be acquired and demonstrated on the playground through the medium of sports.

When I got to sixth grade and learned that we would spend a big chunk of P.E. time doing physical fitness testing, that was a whole different kind of competition, measured against national standards, ranked on a percentile basis, tested against what other girls my age could do. It was the President's Physical Fitness Commission.

Our teacher explained percentiles and informed us that kids who met standards for the 85th percentile would get a cool blue patch with a very presidential eagle. The 80th percentile would get a patch too, though it had a geometric design, no eagle. I wanted the eagle. We did some practice sessions before we did the testing for real, so we could get a sense of where we stood relative to what the president thought we should be able to do. Unfortunately, our first time through the six-minute run made it clear to me that I was not 85th percentile material in distance running. Likewise for the 40-yard dash.

My real downfall, though, was gravity. Gravity took the form of the flexed-arm hang, which was what the president thought that girls should do in place of pull-ups. The flexed-arm hang involved getting up in to the "up" position of a pull-up however you wanted. You could even use a chair. Then you'd hang there with your chin above the bar for as long as you could. Clearly in this faux event, strength was at a premium, which was good, but weight was a disadvantage. My arms wiggled like Jell-O and dropped me on the ground after just a few seconds at the first attempt.

It was time for Plan B. I studied the percentile tables and realized that I had a chance at the second-best patch if I could get my flexed-arm hang up to 17 seconds. The events in 1975 were different from the ones today. I know we had a softball throw, now replaced by a hamstring flexibility test (so weenie), and I think we had a standing broad jump, situps, and pushups.

I had to improve in the 40, probably a second or less, and I also had to run faster over the six minutes, but I had to more than double the amount of time I could hang. My weight was against me, certainly, but my stubbornness and attachment to the patch, even the uglier patch, were on my side. I was coordinated, so I could meet the numbers in the shuttle run, a test of lateral quickness, and another event that involved sideways shuffling between squares. The softball, no worries. Situps and pushups, fine. I think girls got to do girly pushups, our weight resting on our knees. So it was just that whole running and hanging thing that stood in my way.

It's a mystery to me why I wanted the patch so badly that I was willing to spend my own time running around the block at home, doing little sprints down the street, and wrestling my way up to the flexed-arm hang position on top of the swing set bar. I would count one-hippopotamus, two-hippopotamus, three-hippopotamus through clenched teeth, working on the very specific muscle groups needed to keep my chin over the bar for a growing number of hippopotami. As I grimaced and counted, I was aware on one level that this was an extremely foolish activity. However, I was making progress. My hippopotami were multiplying slowly but surely, and soon I was into the double digits in seconds.

The pursuit of the patch didn't seem like drudgery though, even though it might sound like that now. It was work, but it was something I enjoyed for its own sake. Even the endless attempts at flexed-arm hanging.

On the day of the official test for the 40-yard dash I was amped to the gills on adrenaline and raring to go. I can't for the life of me remember what time I needed to get, but when Mr. Newhouse yelled "Go!" I went hell for leather across the blacktop. And I don't know if it was the adrenaline or the sprints down the sidewalk in front of the house, but I sneaked in under the wire exactly on the time I needed. Somehow I struggled to an 80th percentile finish in the six-minute run too, though I have little recollection of the event. It was just running and running and running until I thought I would burst. Mindless endurance, that's all, and for years I disliked distance running for that very reason. It was just about running and suffering, and what was fun about that?

And then came the official test for the flexed-arm hang. I got up on a chair, got over the bar, and hung on for dear life as the seconds counted away. My arms trembled; I gritted my teeth; I raised my chin as high as I could. And then I let go. I hadn't made it. Mr. Newhouse let me try again, but I was tired and I couldn't hold on. I begged him for another few days to practice, and he agreed to wait and send in our results the following week.

I must have spent the whole weekend jumping up onto the swing set, hanging, falling off. I counted 17-hippopotamus a couple of times, but I knew I was counting them as fast as humanly possible. Also, I felt like I got a better grip on the swing set bar, which was thicker and not slippery, than on the pull-up bar at school. But I didn't think I could persuade Mr. Newhouse to come to my house with a stopwatch, so I set up a time with him after school in the playground for the final test of strength. It seemed like such an impossible task, still, after all my practicing, to hold my whole body weight up there for all that time. I felt so heavy, and my arms felt so weak. I heard him say 15, and I hung on for two more hippopotami and then collapsed onto the rubber mat under the bar. Seventeen. A beautiful number, a prime number, the number of my triumph. Mr. Newhouse said, "You know, if you just did a couple more seconds on this, you'd be at the 85th percentile," but I was done. I had worked just about all I could work, and even if I could have done 20 or 21 seconds on the hang, I still would have had to run a lot faster in both the sprint and the long run.

The president's 80th percentile patch, when it finally arrived in a huge and exciting envelope, was definitely not as cool as the eagle patch, but it was huge to my concept of myself as a physical being, as a girl in sports, as an athlete. I learned that I was strong and coordinated compared to other girls my age, and that I could make up for my weaknesses, at least in part, with concerted effort, practice, and sheer stubbornness. But I couldn't make myself run very fast, and I wasn't light.

When you're 10 or 11 or 14 years old, going on a diet to lose a few pounds seems like a fairly easy project. You've never tried this before, but the magazine assures you that it'll be simple and straightforward, and that you'll lose all your unsightly fat in just two weeks. Besides, you're doing it with your mom, so she must know what she's doing, right?

Considering the central role that weight and dieting have played in my life, I find it difficult to believe that I can't remember how old I was when I went on my first diet, but I honestly can't. I must have been in elementary school, but then I can't synch that up with being in any particular grade or with whatever else was going on in my life. How can you be on a diet when you're lunching on greasy cafeteria tacos? Did my mom pack up a brown-bag lunch of cottage cheese and a grapefruit half? Did I diet in the summer, free of the constraints of institutional food?

But more to the point—how can you be on a diet when you're 11? You're just a kid. It's pathetic. You're supposed to be growing. I don't even remember if the first diet was the first go-round of Dr. Atkins low-carb craziness, or whether it was joining Mom's Weight Watchers program. I do remember a period where meat and cheese and mayonnaise were okay, but bread and potatoes were not okay. But I don't remember if that was before or after the time that we had to eat liver once a week. Mom may have asked me if I wanted to join her in a diet. It makes me think that I must have been younger than 12 to have gone along with the plan with such complaisance.

A more perceptive child might have wondered why it used to be good to be a good eater and now it wasn't. Or maybe I didn't need to wonder. Maybe I just knew, from the occasional comments and the frustrating experience of clothes shopping, that dieting was what I was supposed to do.

Dieting didn't even seem hard. The first day you were really hungry, but then on Day Two you'd weigh yourself on the bathroom scale and see that you had already lost 2 of the 10 pounds, and you'd be motivated. You'd eat your grapefruit in the morning; you'd lunch on your tuna with lemon juice; you'd dine on the baked chicken breast with one small potato and a side of green beans—with lemon juice! Mom did the cooking, planning, and shopping. The hunger would get easier after about three days, and pretty soon you'd be down five pounds and Mom would be praising you.

The same mental skills that had served me as a seeker of the president's patch worked to my advantage as a child dieter. I had a good ability to focus on a task, to repeat certain specified activities, and to endure some discomfort and exert effort in pursuit of my objective. It seemed to be easier to lose a few pounds than to learn to hang on a horizontal bar for 17 bloody hippopotami. It was quicker, even if it wasn't a huge amount of fun. I was motivated by the idea of measurable achievement, perhaps even more by praise. At least once during my dieting career Mom paid me a dollar (or more?) for every pound I lost.

Not only don't I remember how old I was, I don't remember how long I was on my first diet or what the diet consisted of. I don't remember how much weight I lost, if any. I don't remember my second diet, or my third. I don't remember if I acquiesced to dieting because I wanted to be thinner or because I knew it would please my mom. Why is it a blur? My battle against my own weight consumed so much of my adolescence and adulthood that I can't understand why that first fateful decision to eat cottage cheese on a bed of lettuce leaves, or whatever the hell it was, has vanished from my mind. Memories of the first diet, a loss of innocence far more terrible than the loss of faith in Santa, seem to have been wiped pretty clean.

I remember a low-carb diet, and I remember following along with Mom's Weight Watchers menus. Weight Watchers in the '70s was a grim deal, and the liver was only part of it. Of course, I remember little except the liver, and so I am greatly indebted to the lovely and talented Wendy McClure for publishing on her website a collection of Weight Watchers recipe cards from 1974, unearthed in her parents' garage.[1] Ms. McClure has preserved for a horrified posterity photos of "Fluffy Mackerel Pudding" and "Melon Mousse," which looks exactly like a butt on a plate. I would rather be hung by my toes for a million hippopotami than try to re-create that recipe.

I got less sporty in high school, a little more alienated. I went out for basketball my freshman year and was doing fine on the frosh-soph team. But one afternoon I was shooting hoops in the driveway and I tweaked my ankle a little. The tweak took weeks to heal, and I couldn't play while I was healing. When the foot finally got better, the coach seemed uninterested in having me come back. I got a little more counterculture and didn't do much in sports, except throw Frisbees around or play some pickup ball with my geek-hippie friends, with occasional bouts of running laps around our half-mile block, late in the evening, when I felt restless.

The diets remained though. Some got pretty extreme, like going two or three days without any caloric intake at all. Somewhere in this period of frequent fasting, I developed my breakfast of champions: a quarter cup of wheat germ mixed with a packet of Sweet-N-Low. Pour boiling water over the whole thing and wait for it to be cool enough to eat. Chew many, many times. Wash down with instant coffee. I dreamed up this breakfast because two or three days of fasting would plug up my colon like a rubber stopper, and I needed to find a way to get things going again, so to speak.

Apparently, they weren't doing all the "good" they should have, because when I went for a physical so I could go work at the library after school, the doctor told me I was in excellent health except for one thing. He cheerfully pointed to his notes. "See what I've written there? 'OBESE'! You should try and lose a few pounds." I was not so counterculture as to question his reasoning, except to wonder, silently, if 5'10" and about 150 really qualified as "OBESE."

The last diet of my high school career was the Scarsdale Diet, which was really famous in the late '70s, first because the book sold well and then because the inventor of the Scarsdale Diet was shot and killed, in Scarsdale itself, by his spurned mistress. It was a big deal in its day. I got it into my head that I wanted to weigh 135 for my college interview. I figured I'd have a better chance of getting into the college of my choice if I was thinner. One of my teachers, who I played basketball with after school sometimes, referred to my regime of tuna packed in water, lettuce, and lemon juice as "making weight," like for a wrestling match or crew. This was the first time that anyone had framed dieting to me in sports terms, like training for a specific event.

That kind of clicked for me—dieting, like sports, had rules and goals. You pushed your body in certain ways to achieve certain results, and if something was hard for you, like the flexed-arm hang or going to bed hungry, you just worked on it until you could do it. If you stopped dieting, or if you stopped training, the skills you needed would get rusty. If you didn't shoot hoops, your jump shot would suffer. If you went off the tuna-and-lettuce path, your skills of denying your appetite would suffer.

I made my weight. I got into Harvard. I very briefly considered rowing, until I found out that the crew worked out at six in the morning. I pretty much gave up dieting, except for a couple of weeks here and there when my best friend and I would eat yogurt for breakfast, salad for lunch, and a hot fudge sundae for dinner.

My senior year, one of my friends had the idea of forming a women's rugby club. Being Welsh, I was all over the idea. I didn't even know that women played rugby, but apparently enough of our fellow students had played in high school that we felt we could have a team. And there were sisters in the art of elegant violence in other schools, so that we could actually have matches. I signed up.

I knew theoretically that rugby involved running, and I hadn't been running much since, well, a long time. I showed up for the first workout in the gym, since it was still too early in the year for outdoor training. We practiced passing the ball backward as we jogged forward; we learned the names of positions and plays, and saw the basic setup of the scrum. That part was all good, but at the end of practice we ran sprints back and forth across the basketball court, and that was less good. I needed some training.

I was extremely motivated. I wanted to catch the ball and plow through a wall of opponents; I wanted to tackle; I wanted to get into the scrum, even after I found out how it worked. So I hit the gym, running on the court, riding the exercise bike, doing some weights. I was on the bike one day when one of my teammates came in and complimented me on my good warm-up. I didn't have the heart to tell her that I wasn't warming up—that was my workout. Still, I made progress in my quest for strong rugby legs and endurance. By the time the snow melted enough to practice outdoors, I thought I could hang.

It turned out "hang" was the operative word. My height and relative lack of speed, coupled with my utter lack of experience, pegged me as a lock forward. My main task was to provide leverage in the scrum. The scrum starts with the hooker, who "hooks" the ball with her feet, putting her arms around the necks of the two props on either side of her. Next, each lock kneels behind the prop forward and the hooker and puts one arm around the other lock, and the other arm up between the legs of the prop in front of her. I'm not making this up. She hangs on to the waistband of the prop's shorts, and when the signal is given to scrum down, all hell breaks loose.

The props and hookers on either side step forward and butt heads with each other, straining to push the other side back and get the ball onto their side. The second row pushes, suspended in an ungainly manner, heads between the butts of the front row, legs pushed out behind, backs flat, and nothing supporting us up front but our arms hanging off the prop in front and the lock on the other side. Hold on too loosely, and you fall on the ground. So you hang on for dear life, and push forward with your legs, and clench your stomach muscles as hard as you can, and then eventually the ball comes out of the scrum, and everyone takes off after it. When this happens, your supports run away from you, and you are left to fall face-first in the mud, with heavy women running over your head and leaving cleat marks on your body. I loved it.

Once we were out on the practice field, I realized that I still wasn't in good enough shape to keep up. It takes a special kind of fitness to push forward as hard as you can in the scrum, fall flat on your face, and then jump up and sprint to tackle someone. With time I got close though, getting out of the mud and up to the action fast enough to make something happen—make a tackle, grab the ball, or get in someone's way. When I got in someone's way, being large was a positive.

The up-and-down life of a lock forward forced me to analyze the advantages and disadvantages of my weight in terms of the sport. For leverage in the scrum, weight was good. Having to support all that weight by hanging off the shorts of the woman in front of me and the woman to my right—less good. For running—not so good. For tackling—good, if I could catch the woman I was aiming for. If I hit someone square on, she would fall down, boom. I liked that. What was really great about being a big strong woman, though, was if I by chance got the ball into my hands, it was near impossible to knock me off my feet.

We hadn't had very many practices before our first match, a road trip out to Holy Cross. We didn't have a real pitch with a 20-meter line (I've spelled it the U.S. way even though it's spelled "metre" when you talk about rugby) or a 50-meter line, or even goalposts. We lined up for the kickoff on what appeared to be a temporarily cowless cow pasture. But I was pumped anyway. I was about to become a rugby player. Roo, who played flanker beside me in the scrum, suffered from trepidation. "We're going to get our bones crushed!" she warbled in tremulous falsetto. "Bones crushed!" I tried to stoke her up by assuring her that it was we who would be crushing the bones of others.

The ladies of Holy Cross were more organized than us, with actual purple rugby jerseys and white shorts. We had a motley collection of shirts, but none of them were purple, so when the ball was kicked off, we knew whose bones to try and crush. I ran down the field in a crimson frenzy, and I remember little else. Toward the end of the match, the ball bounced into my hands around Holy Cross's imaginary 20-meter line. There were no speedy backs around for me to toss the spheroid back to, so I motored forward. I caught my opponents by surprise and managed to gain a good 15 meters before they caught me.

One woman tried to pull me down, then another, but I kept staggering forward. My teammates ran up behind me and "bound on," locking their arms around me and pushing against the opposing tacklers. I held onto the ball like it was made of gold and howled, "Push! PUSH!" We kept moving forward, pushing them toward their own try line. I was surrounded by a heaving mass of sweaty women, half of them grabbing and clawing at the ball, and the other half pushing at my back. I was straining forward, grunting and pushing, and then I could see the line. I don't know how I saw the line because there weren't any lines on the field. Maybe there were some cones. I lunged, quivering with effort, forcing the mass of womanity across the possibly imaginary line. Ha! All I had to do now was touch the ball down to the grass to score the four points. I let my legs go limp and fell with the ball clutched to my chest. Approximately 14 young women, some of them built like me, fell on top of me. The ball contacted my solar plexus with a nauseating impact, and I lay like a beached fish, unable to take a breath, yet filled with fierce triumph.

The referee cleared the bodies away, and after a horrifying few seconds, my diaphragm regained the ability to move. I had scored a try, and the match was over. I was a lock forward, and I had scored a try. I was big and strong, and that was why I had scored. If I was small, I wouldn't have gotten anywhere near the try line, and moreover, I would have gotten my bones crushed. I was proud.

So it's complicated. My cycles of dieting, sportiness, training, being casually or seriously insulted for my weight, injuries, relative indolence, and back to some sport continued throughout my adult life. Some rugby at Berkeley, an injury playing Frisbee, years without sports except for darts, a bout with NutriSystems and fairly serious running, up to 10k for the first time. Being told I might be perceived as too fat to go on a rafting expedition to Siberia, even though I was the only person in the organization who actually spoke Russian. Holding my own in the whitewater and with the attendant camping and hiking. More rounds of dieting, walking to lose weight, then running and swimming and cycling to lose weight—but also because I loved the movement, loved to be physical, loved to be strong and push my body. The running and swimming and cycling led to short and then long triathlons, half marathons, a marathon. A period of less active training and no dieting, the pattern of regaining weight. A period of more training and weight gain. Going to a doctor after a five-day backpacking trip and being asked, "Do you do any exercise?" A period of severe physical debility, tentatively diagnosed, finally, as chronic fatigue/immune dysfunction syndrome.

During months of forced inactivity, where even a walk to the mailbox made my muscles burn and twitch and my joints ache, I yearned for the ability to go for a walk or a bike ride. I pined for the feel of a good tired, the tired when your muscles have worked a good amount and want to rest.

And finally, finally, the decision not to diet anymore, ever. Not to be better at sports, not to fit into some size clothes, or to fit into a definition of acceptable sizes for a woman. To just live, to be the size that I am, and to take care of my body the best I can, as the person I am.

I am a woman who is fat and strong and no longer apologetic. I like to be outside and move my body, but I don't get to it every single day. Sometimes I'm injured. Sometimes I'm tired or grumpy or feel like watching TV. Some days I eat food with lots of sugar in it; some days I eat salad because I want a salad. I'm still figuring out to what degree I actually like vegetables. My relationship to them was ruined by years of dieting, and I'm repairing it, slowly, inconsistently. I don't eat competitively and I don't diet, competitively or otherwise.

I have participated in a few athletic events since I gave up dieting and became a confirmed fatty. An organized bike ride, a couple of short triathlons, part of a marathon relay. The last couple of years, not even that. Maybe I will again.

But a few days ago, I got a wetsuit in the mail. I ordered it made to my own particular measurements. I live at the beach now, but the water's too cold to swim in without a neoprene superhero suit. So I got a neoprene superhero suit.

And a used longboard. And before summer is done I just might be the fattest surfer at my beach. And because I'm fat, I will float easily and stay warm in my wetsuit for a long time.

And I will be proud, and happy. If that's a disease, American Medical Association, then my advice to you is to fuck right the way off. That is the Body Impolitic.

NOTE

1. http://www.candyboots.com.

9

I Know It Wasn't the Fish: Fat in the Consulting Room

Cheryl L. Fuller

I don't know who discovered water, but I know it wasn't the fish.
— Marshall McLuhan

I thought that until I spoke no one would notice me when I entered a room. I could imagine being Echo, the voice without a body. I could wrap myself in my invisibility cloak of charm and move through the world insulated from the judgments and scrutiny of others. It was simply too painful for me to consider the absurdity of that belief; had I done so, I wouldn't have gone anywhere. I now know that long before I say a word, when I walk into a room people see me and will have judgments, fantasies, and beliefs about me based purely on my size. I might wish otherwise but I know that to be so. Samantha Murray, a fat studies scholar, describes what it is like to be subjected to the medical gaze:[1]

> I stand before you now, and I can feel you all "knowing" my body. You see my fatness, and co-extensive with it, you perceive its indisputable deviation from practices of health and care of the body. I am aware that here, in this space, in fact in most spaces, my body is a quintessential symbol of pathology. When you witness me now: seeing my dimpled thighs, my soft bulges and fatty rolls, you believe you know me. The visible marker of my fatness is laden with knowledges of who I am. Looking at me now, you must ask yourself what you know about my body, and, therefore, about me? The visible markers of my fatness, my wide hips, protruding belly, vast thighs, all signal a knowingness of pathology and disease. You read my fat as symptomatic of overeating, lack of exercise, poor nutrition. You see me as a high-risk candidate for diabetes, gall bladder disease, hypertension and heart attack. At a deeper level, you

may see a lazy woman without willpower, a sedentary being, a woman out of control, a woman of unmanaged desires and gluttonous obsessions.[2]

As a woman who has been fat since childhood, I have a long history of struggling with feeling seen as fat before and often instead of being seen as a woman, or a person—of experiencing that gaze, a thin gaze. Several times in my life I have sought therapy only to find myself on the defensive about my body and my weight and without regard for what I felt or wanted. Those experiences, then being told that my weight would likely disqualify me for training as a Jungian analyst, fed an anger that I all too seldom expressed or even allowed into my awareness.

The effect of that gaze, which is always present, is that the woman's own gaze, the way she sees herself, echoes that of the culture and she "ruthlessly evaluates her own body as ruthlessly as she expects to be evaluated."[3] Every time I saw a new therapist—and over the course of my lifetime I have seen five for more than a session or two—I encountered that gaze, and with it the assumption that I should want to lose weight. Even a therapist who was himself fat worked from the assumption that I should want to lose weight. Otherwise, he wondered, how could I ever feel desirable? Eventually, I became able to use anger to defend myself, which, of course, only made me come across as defensive, but at least that was better than mutely accepting their indictment. But inside, under the anger, I felt shame and pain.

Soon after Irvin Yalom published his book *Love's Executioner*, I began working with a new analyst, a man. One piece in particular, "Fat Lady," bothered me and surfaced all of my anxieties about working in analysis with a man, a slender attractive man. In that piece, Yalom tells of his work with Betty, a fat woman. I recoiled in horror at what he wrote:

> The day Betty entered my office, the instant I saw her steering her ponderous two-hundred-fifty-pound, five-foot-two-inch frame toward my trim, high-tech office chair, I knew that a great trial of countertransference was in store for me.
>
> I have always been repelled by fat women. I find them disgusting: their absurd sidewise waddle, their absence of body contour, breasts, laps, buttocks, shoulders, jawlines, cheekbones, everything, everything I like to see in a woman, obscured in an avalanche of flesh. And I hate their clothes, the shapeless, baggy dresses or, worse, the stiff elephantine blue jeans with the barrel thighs. How dare they impose that body on the rest of us? . . .
>
> Of course, I am not alone in my bias. Cultural reinforcement is everywhere. Who ever has a kind word for the fat lady? But my contempt

surpasses all cultural norms. Early in my career, I worked in a maximum security prison where the least heinous offense committed by any of my patients was a simple, single murder. Yet I had little difficulty accepting those patients, attempting to understand them, and finding ways to be supportive.

But when I see a fat lady eat, I move down a couple of rungs on the ladder of human understanding. I want to tear the food away. To push her face into the ice cream. "Stop stuffing yourself! Haven't you had enough, for Chrissakes?," I'd like to wire her jaws shut!

Poor Betty, thank God, thank God, knew none of this as she innocently continued her course toward my chair, slowly lowered her body, arranged her folds and, with her feet not quite reaching the floor, looked up at me expectantly.[4]

Was that what my analyst was feeling as he sat across from me? I felt self-conscious before entering the room where we met. I remember copying the essay and giving it to him to read. I wanted him to see how awful Yalom's attitude was and hoped he would tell me he was not like that. I wanted to ask him if he shared Yalom's views, but when I tried, the words would not come. So long as I was in the grip of the gaze, what he felt hardly mattered because I had internalized it to the point that I was my own overseer.

There is no question that openly admitting such strong prejudice, such clear countertransference, as Yalom did, takes some courage. Then again, it is acceptable to hate fat and to think ill of fat people, so there was little chance of serious criticism except from the fat acceptance community, who could be dismissed as defensive. Nevertheless, I do hand it to him for saying out loud what I am quite certain many therapists feel and never speak. What I feared my own analyst felt.

The essay goes on to talk about the process of therapy, of Betty's depression, and her weight loss, which by the time treatment ends amounts to 100 pounds. And of course the consensus is that because she lost so much weight, this therapy was spectacularly successful. At the end of the essay, Yalom writes:

"It's the same with me, Betty. I'll miss our meetings. But I'm changed as a result of knowing you ."

She had been crying, her eyes downcast, but at my words she stopped sobbing and looked toward me, expectantly.

"And, even though we won't meet again, I'll still retain that change."

"What change?"

"Well, as I mentioned to you, I hadn't had much professional experience with the problem of obesity." I noted Betty's eyes drop with disappointment and silently berated myself for being so impersonal.

"Well, what I mean is that I hadn't worked before with heavy patients, and I've gotten a new appreciation for the problems of." I could see from her expression that she was sinking even deeper into disappointment. "What I mean is that my attitude about obesity has changed a lot. When we started I personally didn't feel comfortable with obese people." In unusually feisty terms, Betty interrupted me. "Ho! ho! ho! Didn't feel comfortable. That's putting it mildly. Do you know that for the first six months you hardly ever looked at me? And in a whole year and a half you've never, not once, touched me? Not even for a handshake!"

My heart sank. My God, she's right! I have never touched her. I simply hadn't realized it. And I guess I didn't look at her very often either. I hadn't expected her to notice![5]

How naive for Yalom to think that Betty hadn't known all along of his distaste. Having lived in a world of people who shared his feelings of disgust, she was an expert at detecting it and doing what she could to minimize herself as a target for their scorn. And in her rebuke, she points out that in fact he has changed far less than he imagines.

I wonder what Betty is like now, more than 30 years later. The chances are very good that she has gained back all 100 pounds and maybe more, because that's what happens with repeated dieting as, in a cruel slap at the efforts to tame the flesh, each diet leads to gaining back more than was lost. Or maybe she has now had bariatric surgery. Or perhaps she is in that tiny minority who succeeded in maintaining weight loss. But no one ever questioned why she would lose weight and what the effect of a therapist filled with contempt and disgust for her body would have on her feelings about herself. If even your therapist finds you repulsive, what hope is there after all?

How is a fat person, who, no matter the reasons for being fat, certainly has a whole host of emotional issues about her size and her body—how is such a person to find the courage to talk about those feelings in the presence of someone who finds her as disgusting as she herself often does? How can she give voice to her anger at the prejudice she encounters? How is she to arrive at being able to care about her body and for herself lovingly rather than with contempt and hatred? And what happens if she doesn't want to devote herself to losing all that weight? Supposing she wants to get off the diet merry-go-round and concentrate on being healthy and fat?

In the Jungian world we speak of complexes. A complex is an emotionally charged group of ideas or images. When an individual or group is in the grip of a complex, their vision is distorted by the ideas and images of the complex. A person caught in a complex has a "sore spot," which leads to behavior that is automatic and stereotypical. The same response appears in every triggering situation, whether it is appropriate and helpful or not.

Complexes exist on the individual level, and they also exist in groups. Such complexes are called "cultural complexes":

> Intense collective emotion is the hallmark of an activated cultural complex at the core of which is an archetypal pattern. Cultural complexes structure emotional experience and operate in the personal and collective psyche in much the same way as individual complexes, although their content might be quite different. Like individual complexes, cultural complexes tend to be repetitive, autonomous, resist consciousness, and collect experience that confirms their historical point of view. And, as already mentioned, cultural complexes tend to be bipolar, so that when they are activated, the group ego or the individual ego of a group member becomes identified with one part of the unconscious cultural complex, while the other part is projected out onto the suitable hook of another group or one of its members. Individuals and groups in the grips of a particular cultural complex automatically take on a shared body language and postures or express their distress in similar somatic complaints. Finally, like personal complexes, cultural complexes can provide those caught in their potent web of stories and emotions a simplistic certainty about the group's place in the world in the face of otherwise conflicting and ambiguous uncertainties.[6]

Our culture is in the grip of a fat complex, which takes its most obvious form in the so-called war on obesity.

Consider the views of Kathy Leach, a practitioner of transactional analysis in the UK, which she sets out in her book, *The Overweight Patient: A Psychological Approach to Understanding and Working with Obesity*. The book opens pretty well—

> In the light of recent growing emphasis on what has become known as the "great weight debate", I believe that it must be understood that if it were easy to lose weight then sufferers (for that is what these patients are) of obesity would lose weight rather than face the ridicule, non-acceptance and feelings of shame resulting from their size. This book offers a way of understanding the psychological aspects of the problem that prevents people from losing weight or maintaining weight loss.[7]

She seems get it but then things go awry:

> There are two major clinical concerns, both of which are addressed in this book. They are:

1. That there are two aspects of maintaining a large body size: the need to eat excess food and the need to be fat. These are two separate, albeit related, issues. What this means is that, if the patient psychologically needs her large body size then attention focused only on her eating and feeding non-biological needs with food will be ineffective. The therapist needs to enable the patient to discover the meaning of, and reasons for, her protective body armouring. These patients will undoubtedly also be using food to feed psychological needs, but attention to both aspects is necessary for the patient to change.

2. That there are differences in the defensive structure of the patient who has been overweight for a shorter length of time or is in the lower half of the obese to morbidly obese index compared with the long-term or lifelong sufferer or morbidly obese patient. The therapeutic direction and the availability of the patient to work with cognition (thinking) and affect (feelings) will differ depending on the length of time the patient has been overweight.[8]

In my own clinical experience I have found that maintaining overweight and overeating are survival decisions. That is to say, the patient has an unconscious belief (until brought into awareness) that she will not survive unless she overeats or remains obese.[9]

And here we are again in the same old blame game where the fat person is responsible for being fat and is wearing her irresponsibility right there in her body for all to see. If only she would straighten out her thinking, life would change.

I am working to find out why the patient needs to maintain a large size or to eat excessively. I do not work towards weight loss as the primary goal, I aim to treat the cause not the symptom and so I aim/encourage the patient to understand why she needs the food or the weight and what options are open to her to address these reasons. My goal is for the patient to have a choice about her weight loss and that genuine psychological and social choice comes from knowing why she has needed to overeat or be big in the world in order to cope.[10]

In the universe of psychotherapists, I locate myself among the Jungians. Though I wish it otherwise, I have no reason to assume that the Jungian world is any freer of this fat complex than the rest of the healing professions. I am puzzled nonetheless by the silence in the Jungian literature about obesity. There are books and articles about anorexia but not about fat, not about obesity. Much is made of the need to connect with the body, of the body as storehouse of memory. *Quadrant's* description says it is a journal of "essays grounded in personal and professional experience, which focus on issues of matter and body, psyche and spirit."[11] Yet there are no articles that I can find about fat, save for one four years ago, "The Epidemic of Obesity in Contemporary American Culture: A Jungian Reflection,"[12] which focuses on compulsive eating. Again fat is equated with gluttony. There is nothing about fat in the 50-plus year archives of the *Journal of Analytical Psychology*. In what used to be the *San Francisco Library Journal* and is now the *Jung Journal: Culture & Psyche*, there are two interviews with Marion Woodman, in which some of her thoughts about fat are offered, and reviews of her two books that dealt with fat and anorexia. And that is it. Heuer notes, "Jungian psychology seems marked by a theoretical ambivalence towards the body, whilst mostly ignoring it clinically ... so the post-Jungians have only rarely engaged with the body in their theoretical and clinical work."[13] Or as Jung put it:

> We do not like to look at the shadow-side of ourselves; therefore there are many people in civilized society who have lost their shadow altogether, have lost the third dimension, and with it they have usually lost the body. The body is a most doubtful friend because it produces things we do not like: there are too many things about the personification of this shadow of the ego. Sometimes it forms the skeleton in the cupboard, and everybody naturally wants to get rid of such a thing.[14]

Could it be that the assumption that fat is a symptom of underlying conflict and complexes is so deep and automatic that it seems unquestionable, not worthy of examination? Is it disgust, as we saw in Yalom with Betty or as Miller wonders in relation to homosexuality:

> It is useful to reflect upon how disgust is dealt with in an analytic situation ... Does the analyst relate to disgust as something to be overcome or something to penetrate more deeply? Can the analyst tolerate disgust about a racial type, a form of sexual expression, unwanted desires, or even certain ideas? Is the analytic work inclined toward the dissolution of this disgust or the pursuit of its use in the life of an individual? ... The possibility here is that a contemporary psychotherapist might react to the disgust ... by seeing it as something to be overcome rather than finding its relevance or purpose to his life. It is at these intersections that the analyst is challenged to separate his or her own values and goals from the process of the other individual, the analysand, who has another agenda for these feelings and attitudes.[15]

My first analyst was a woman. I chose her because at the time, she was the only Jungian analyst within reasonable driving distance of where I lived. I was

40 with two children and an unhappy marriage. I had been in therapy before, most recently for three years with a charismatic and difficult man. I had in mind that I would someday like to pursue Jungian analytic training, but that was not my primary reason for seeing her. It was that I was 40 and I knew I needed to deal with what I wanted in my life in the years ahead. She was slender and very well dressed, the kind of woman with whom I often felt clumsy and ungainly. At the beginning I said something to her to the effect that the issue of my weight was nonnegotiable, a stance occasioned in large measure because of her resemblance to my mother and because I had worked so hard through my thirties to make peace with my body, to stop dieting and hating myself for being fat. In spite of that declaration or maybe because of it, after a couple of sessions, she told me of a dream she had had when she was in analysis, a dream she had had, she believed, for her analyst who, like me, was fat. In the dream, Jung told her that "every extra ounce costs a pound of consciousness." She told me her analyst had been grateful to her for telling her and had undertaken to lose weight because of it. I was not grateful. Not at all. I was angry and hurt that she had so clearly not heard me when I said I was not willing to make weight loss a focus of my work with her. I know I wrote to her about my anger but I also know that my expression of it was pretty impotent. I wanted her to be willing to see me as I was, to sit with me as I was and allow me to open up to her, and to myself, about my experience in my body, in my life. I needed to be able to speak and be heard without the blame that comes with the belief that all I had to do to be "normal" was to eat less and move more. But that was not to be.

She wanted me to read and talk with her about an English fairy tale, "The Laidly Worm of Spindleston Heugh,"[16] a tale she connected to hunger and the mother complex. I read it. But by then I was armored against her and did not trust her enough to allow myself to explore with her the issues of my body, hunger, my mother, and my weight. Still she did not give up and asked if I wouldn't consider losing a few pounds. I was furious at the suggestion. How many pounds would be enough? Why should I step again into that madness of dieting and food obsession and anger and depression? And why would I deliberately put myself again in the position of seeing the loss, so hard fought for, disappear as the pounds came back, as they always did? She had no answer. We did not talk about it again in the three years I worked with her. And I am sorry to say I never dealt with how I felt about her. In fact I left that analysis without closure on that issue.

As soon as that analyst inserted her agenda about my weight, she became another in the long line of people in my life who had attempted to shame, cajole, or otherwise make me diet and cede control of what I ate to someone or something else. In relating her dream to me, she was telling me that she believed that every extra ounce of weight cost me a pound of consciousness.

And further, because she herself was quite slender, that she had not suffered that penalty and thus was superior to me. For her, it was more important that I be willing to lose weight than that she listen to my experience and feelings about being fat. And when she did that, her countertransference, fully in synch with the cultural attitude, met my internalized loathing of my body and fat and served only to push me away from her. I could not risk talking about what it is like to be fat, to live under that gaze, to feel the judgment and disgust that is part of the everyday life of fat people. "A fat body is cruelly stigmatized in this culture. It is treated, seen, felt as the object of disgust and fear. Many disabilities are so treated and seen; but fatness is also seen as reason to blame the fat person who ate his or her way into 'freakishness.' "[17]

For that analyst, as for Yalom, it was a given that my fat was something that must be eradicated. All of the cultural notions about fat—the disgust, the belief that it represented unbridled appetite, and all of the other common cultural stereotypes—are part of the background of belief, unexamined and often unconscious for them, and indeed for most therapists and others in helping professions, gripped as they by our culture's fat complex.[18]

> It is the beliefs which are so much a matter of course that they are rather tacitly presupposed than formally expressed and argued for, the ways of thinking which seem so natural and inevitable that they are not scrutinized with the eye of logical self-consciousness, that often are the most decisive of the character of a philosopher's doctrine, and still oftener of the dominant intellectual tendencies of an age.[19]

That is how Lovejoy described the kind of climate in which we now live. Or, as McLuhan more succinctly put it, "I don't know who discovered water, but I know it wasn't the fish." We fish swim in this sea of judgment and disgust and hatred of fat, as if fat were itself a source of evil in the world. It is so much a part of our culture that it is a given. Only that minority of people who are fat activists or otherwise involved with body diversity and/or the Health at Every Size movement along with a few researchers are even aware of the water in which we swim.

It seems that most therapists, along with the people we encounter everywhere every day, assume that fat people eat gluttonously—huge portions of high-fat sugary "unhealthy" foods like piles of doughnuts, mammoth plates of pasta, a whole pizza—because how else could they have become fat, if not from gorging themselves on any and all food available to them? They seem unable to imagine a fat person choosing a salad or for that matter a slender person gorging himself on ice cream or a huge burger. It is not possible to determine how or what a person eats by looking at her.

> Therapists are easily or subtly prey to the cultural mandates for the female body ... This mandate is... fat phobic, obsessed with bodily

control, in revolt against aging and it's concomitant bodily changes, out-
raged at and contemptuous of the imperfect out-of-control body and
repulsed by immodest female appetites and hunger.[20]

There is very little written about body meeting body in psychotherapy of
any kind. When patient and therapist sit down together, they are meeting
body to body as well as mind to mind. And each brings with her all of her
assumptions, feelings, and projections about bodies, both her own and that
of the other. In the case of dealing with fat patients, it seems more than usually
important for the therapist to be aware of her own attitudes and complexes
around weight and appearance:

> In examining one's countertransference responses to obese patients in
> psychotherapy, it is important to note that the obese patient's appear-
> ance may actually be repulsive, distorting the human physique to grotes-
> que proportions . . . Therapists should intermittently ask themselves how
> they feel about their patients' obesity and how they have minimized or
> exaggerated the meaning of the patients' excess weight. If in the course
> of therapy, the patients' obesity is to be discussed or if it is discussed to
> the exclusion of other issues, therapists should examine their counter-
> transference responses as well as the patients' resistances.[21]

I have taught my analyst about the water we swim in. In an article he wrote
some years ago, he said of me, "Her weight belies her intelligence." When he
gave me the article to read to see if I was okay with it, I was furious and hurt.
When I read it, that phrase confirmed all of my fears about how he viewed me.
We have discussed that phrase many times since then. He now says it was a
ridiculous thing to say, but when he wrote it, gripped by the cultural fat complex, he couldn't see the absurdity of what he was saying. In the territory of the
complex, of course one would not expect a fat woman to also be intelligent,
because if she were intelligent she wouldn't be so fat.

Being as he is a naturally slender man, he has had difficulty understanding
the differences in the experience of the world for a fat person from his as a
slender person. Thin privilege has created blindness. For some time I lay on
the couch during my sessions. His couch groaned, literally, under me. Every
time I lay on it, I tensed, fearing this would be the time it would break. It is
a fat person's nightmare to even imagine a piece of furniture breaking under-
neath her weight. When I wanted to use it again after a period away from it,
he told me that it wouldn't hold me. Was it me? Had I somehow in the
months since last I lay on it become too big, too heavy in some way not measurable? Or had it simply broken down from use? Why have it if it could not
hold me? I was humiliated, furious when I was told I was too much for the

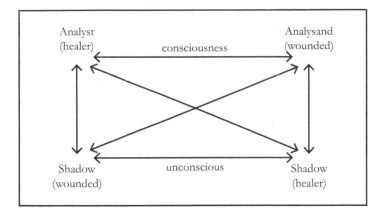

Figure 9.1 Effects of therapy on both therapist and patient in Jungian belief.

couch. I wanted him to fix it, to know that he was rejecting me by having a couch that couldn't hold me. I felt as if the space that could hold all of me shrank.

In the Jungian environment, the belief is that not only the patient but also the therapist is changed in the process of the therapy, which is to say that the patient on an unconscious level functions as therapist to the unconscious patient in the therapist, illustrated in Figure 9.1.[22]

This is not the prevailing view in most types of therapy today, where the expert/therapist offers techniques to the patient who will then change. But when it works, when patient and therapist are able to influence each other, both do change. In the case of dealing with fat, usually it would be a fat patient free enough of the cultural fat complex, a fish able to see the water, who can insist that losing weight is not the solution to her problems and who can dare to confront her therapist's attitudes and beliefs.

Last year "the U.S. Preventive Services Task Force urged doctors to iden-tify patients with a body mass index of 30 or more and either provide counsel-ing themselves or refer the patient to a program designed to promote weight loss and improve health prospects . . . These programs would set weight-loss goals, improve knowledge about nutrition, teach patients how to track their eating and set limits, identify barriers to change (such as a scarcity of healthful food choices near home) and strategize on ways to maintain lifestyle changes."[23] Around the same time the American Psychological Association issued a call for a panel to develop guidelines to "address the problem of obesity":

For much of the population, obesity is associated with disease and mor-tality. It can be effectively treated through behavior change, which falls within the domain of psychologists. As collaborations between psychologists and other healthcare professionals increase, psychologists are expected to be called upon more frequently to address obesity and other physical conditions.[24]

There is no call for polling or surveying fat people to see what we might want. There is no recognition of the fact that there is no evidence that obesity can be effectively treated through behavioral change. There is no such treatment and all treatments thus far, regardless of modality, have at best a 90 to 95 percent failure rate.[25] No concern is raised about the ethics of promoting treatments that fail the vast majority of the time and thus are likely to only increase the sense of failure and stigma so many fat patients already feel.

I don't know what would bring about the kind of change needed for it to become the norm, rather than the exception, for a fat therapy patient to be perceived as a patient who should be asked what she wants to work on, for her not to be subject to the suggestion that she could/should lose at least a little weight, for it to enter the mind of the therapist that this patient may not see her weight as the problem in her life, even though she experiences the negative effects of stigma and bias. The operative assumption is that in a room with a normal-weight therapist and a fat patient, it is the patient who has a weight problem. In a little book published in the late '80s, *Fat Oppression and Psychotherapy*, Laura Brown puts her finger on a problem: "While it was acceptable for clients to be fat women, therapists as so-called models of good functioning, we're required to stay thin."[26]

Someone said that we fat people have not yet had our Stonewall moment, where a critical mass of fat people becomes aware of the cultural complex operating against them and rises to make a noise loud enough to penetrate the complex and begin to weaken its grip. Until that moment, we make headway case by case.

NOTES

1. Foucault coined the term "medical gaze" to denote the dehumanizing medical separation of the patient's body from the patient's person.

2. Samantha Murray as quoted in Michael Gard and Jan Wright, *The Obesity Epidemic: Science, Morality and Ideology* (New York: Routledge, 2005), 166.

3. Jana Evans Braziel and Kathleen LeBesco, eds., *Bodies Out of Bounds* (Berkeley: University of California Press, 2005), 62.

4. Irvin D. Yalom, *Love's Executioner, and Other Tales of Psychotherapy* (New York: Harper Perennial, 1990), 94–95.

5. Ibid., 123.

6. Thomas Singer and Samuel L. Kimbles, eds., *The Cultural Complex*, Kindle ed. (Hove, UK: Brunner-Routledge, 2004), 6.

7. Kathy Leach, *The Overweight Patient: A Psychological Approach to Understanding and Working with Obesity* (Philadelphia: Jessica Kingsley, 2006), 9.

8. Ibid., 10–11.

9. Ibid., 13.

10. Ibid., 14.

11. *Quadrant,* published by the New York Jung Foundation, is one of the major Jungian journals.

12. *Quadrant: The Journal of the C. G. Jung Foundation* 39, no. 1 (Winter 2009).

13. Gerhard Heuer, " 'In My Flesh I Shall See God': Jungian Body Psychotherapy," in *New Dimensions in Body Psychotherapy*, ed. N. Totton (New York: Open University Press, 2005), 107.

14. C. G. Jung, *Analytical Psychology: Its Theory and Practice* (New York: Vintage Press, 1968), 23.

15. Barry Miller, "Expressions of Homosexuality and the Perspective of Analytical Psychology," *Journal of Analytical Psychology* 55 (2010): 116.

16. The text of this fairy tale can be found here: http://www.surlalunefairytales.com/authors/jacobs/english/laidlyworm.html, as accessed on March 15, 2013.

17. Carol Bloom et al., eds., *Eating Problems: A Feminist Psychoanalytic Treatment Model* (New York: Basic Books, 1994), 154.

18. As reported by NAAFA, the National Association to Advance Fat Acceptance, the Rudd Center at Yale found:

"In a study of 400 doctors:

1 out of 3 listed obesity as a condition to which they respond negatively, ranked behind only drug addiction, alcoholism, and mental illness.

Obesity was associated with noncompliance, hostility, dishonesty, & poor hygiene

Self-report studies show that doctors view obese patients as lazy, lacking in self-control, non-compliant, unintelligent, weak-willed, and dishonest

Psychologists ascribe more pathology, more negative and severe symptoms, and worse prognosis to obese patients compared to thinner patients presenting identical psychological profiles"

http://www.naafaonline.com/dev2/the_issues/health.html (accessed May 17, 2014), based on: http://www.yaleruddcenter.org/resources/upload/docs/what/reports/RuddBriefWeightBias2009.pdf.

19. Arthur Oncken Lovejoy, *The Great Chain of Being: A Study of the History of an Idea* (Cambridge, MA: Harvard University Press, 1976), 7.

20. Susan Gutwil in, Bloom et al., 152.

21. William K. Drell, "Countertransference and the Obese Patient," *American Journal of Psychotherapy* 42, no. 1 (January 1988): 79.

22. C. G. Jung, adapted from *The Psychology of the Transference*, Collected Works, vol. 16 (Princeton, NJ: Princeton University Press, 1966), para. 422.

23. See http://www.latimes.com/news/nationworld/nation/la-sci-obesity-screening-20120622,0,2815818.story.

24. See http://www.apa.org/science/about/psa/2012/04/obesity-ptsd.aspx.

25. T. Mann et al., "Medicare's Search for Effective Obesity Treatments: Diets Are Not the Answer," *American Psychologist* 62, no. 3 (April 2007): 220–33.

26. Laura Brown, *Fat Oppression and Psychotherapy: A Feminist Perspective* (New York: Haworth Press, 1989).

10

Body Shaming, Binge Eating Disorder, and Fat Acceptance

Ashley Ruiz-Margenot

The first time I remember being aware of my eating disorder, I was about 10 years old. I was sitting in my middle school guidance class, learning about eating disorders. My teacher, Ms. Hollowell, stood at the front of the room telling us about anorexia and bulimia: what we should look for, what the signs were, what it would do to our bodies. I sat there, feeling uncomfortable. I could relate to what she was saying about people with these eating disorders, but the criteria she presented did not entirely fit me.

I understood bingeing. By this point in my life, it was a part of my routine to stash food in my room and eat it when I was alone. Food was my secret love. Sneaking it out of the kitchen was a top-secret operation that required a great deal of skill and stealth. I also understood restricting food, to some extent, although it took me more than a decade after this classroom lecture to see the role it played in my life. I sat in the classroom wondering if there was a place in this discussion for someone like me. I had not stopped eating altogether, but I was on self-imposed restrictive diets all the time. I was not purging, but I was bingeing.

At some point in the lecture, I decided to raise my hand and ask the question: "Is there an eating disorder where people binge but don't purge?" My teacher thought for a moment.

"Yes, that's something," she said, and went back to her lesson.

I look back on that day in school more than I care to admit. I replay that day in my mind and I wonder what path my life would have taken had my teacher known to say, "That's an eating disorder, too." At the time, we did not have the knowledge we have today about binge eating disorder, or BED. It was not until 2013 that BED was included as a separate eating disorder with its own diagnostic criteria in the newest edition of the *Diagnostic and Statistical*

Manual of Mental Disorders (DSM-V).[1] The previous edition, the *DSM-IV*, included only three diagnostic categories for eating disorders: anorexia nervosa, bulimia nervosa, and eating disorders not otherwise specified (EDNOS). For those with BED, this meant being lumped into the EDNOS category, if the disorder was recognized at all. Today, it is recognized as "the most common eating disorder in the United States, affecting 3.5% of women and 2% of men," according to the Binge Eating Disorder Association. The National Institute of Diabetes and Digestive and Kidney Diseases estimates that two out of three people with BED are obese.[2] However, this does not mean that all fat individuals have this disorder, nor can you diagnose an eating disorder by the size of a person's body.

The *DSM-V* outlines the following criteria for BED:[3]

- Episodes of binge eating that occur at least once a week for a period of at least three months
- Eating a larger amount of food than is normal in a short time frame (what constitutes this amount depends on the individual)
- Lack of control over eating during binge episodes; a feeling that one cannot control what or how much he or she is eating, and that she or he cannot stop

So what makes a binge, a binge? The *DSM-V* also provides some guidance in this area:

- Eating until feeling uncomfortably full
- Eating large amounts of food when not physically hungry
- Eating much more quickly than is normal
- Eating alone out of embarrassment
- Feeling ashamed of these binge episodes

According to the Binge Eating Disorder Association, it is also important to note that there are other criteria that distinguish BED from other eating disorders. Unlike bulimia, a person with BED does not engage in behaviors to "compensate" for their binges, such as purging or excessive exercise. The *DSM-V* also states that people with BED experience "marked distress regarding binge eating."

Before I sought help for my eating disorder, I experienced every one of these symptoms. I was ashamed of my relationship with food. I had a habit of sneaking food out of my parents' kitchen and bringing it into my room to eat by myself. I would ride my bike to the local convenience store to buy more food, which was against my parents' rule of staying inside our neighborhood and away from busy streets. I found out at a young age that living with my eating disorder meant breaking a lot of rules and crossing lines I never dreamed I would cross.

My bunk bed provided the perfect hiding place for my food. A hole in the box spring of the top bunk held my secret stash. When I was alone at night, or home alone in the house, I would choose that moment to eat. Food was a source of comfort for me. If I was lonely, food was my friend and confidante. If I was angry, food calmed me down. If I was sad, food made me happy. To me, food seemed like the ultimate friend because it did not judge me and would always be available. Food was never too busy for me, and I found myself making time to spend with the food that I was hiding from everyone.

I became an expert in covering up my binges. I rearranged the trash to hide any suspicious candy wrappers or pizza boxes. Sometimes I threw them out in a dumpster down the street to avoid suspicion. What I could not cover up, however, was how my body had changed in response to my binge eating. My parents, not knowing about the binges, could not understand how I was suddenly gaining weight. My doctor was equally perplexed. I remember one doctor's appointment when the doctor announced that I had gained about eight pounds since the last visit, only a few months before. My parents were stunned. On the previous doctor's appointment, I had actually lost weight. Now I had gained it all back and then some.

"Well, someone must be bringing food into the house!" the doctor said accusatorily. I sat on the exam table, feeling humiliated and guilty. No one knew my secret, and it would be another 13 years before my parents would find out that I spent a large percentage of my childhood and teenage years binge eating and restricting food under their roof. I began to try and counteract the binges with diets.

Before I ever tried any commercial diet plan, I put myself on one. I marked days on my calendar when I was supposed to eat healthy and days when I was allowed to binge. I marked the latter with the word "pig," short for "pig out." I spent time in my room at night before bed exercising to my Disney cassette tapes. For weights, I used school textbooks. I was convinced this could help me. I would lose weight and no one would ever have to look at me in that shaming, accusatory way ever again. I could take control.

Of course, my eating disorder got worse before it could ever get better. From the time it began at the age of nine, I had problems with my weight. I kept gaining and I could not stop it, because I could not stop bingeing. Eating an entire pizza by myself, eating constantly when I was alone, began to show on my body. Instead of seeing someone who needed help, however, many people saw a girl who needed a diet. I was made fun of in school by my peers. Going to the doctor became a source of pain and anxiety for me, as it still is today. Just about every time I came in for an appointment, I had gained weight. At no point did anyone ask me about eating disordered behaviors, or even inquire if there was something going on in my life that would cause this kind of eating or weight gain. Instead, it was an inquisition. Where was this weight coming from? Why couldn't I stop it? What was I doing wrong?

When my guidance counselor started talking about eating disorders that day in class, I thought I had my answer. In the years between the start of my eating disorder and finding recovery, I often had the sneaking suspicion that I had a problem that went beyond the type of food or amount I was eating. I believed I had an eating disorder, but at the same time I could not conceive of the idea that a girl like me could have such a problem. I thought eating disorders happened to thin, white girls. As a fat Latina girl, I did not fit the mold. I was not thin enough. I did not restrict enough. I believed I was teetering on the edge of the eating disorder pool, and the only thing that kept me from diving in was the erroneous belief that I would have to stop eating entirely to have a "real" eating disorder. My mind often told me that this was something I could aspire to, if only I had the willpower.

I struggled for years before a seemingly innocuous project in graduate school opened my eyes. I was in an addictions counseling class, and it was time to start the project that had become a bit famous in our program. I had to give up something I could scarcely live without for six weeks. All around the room, people were giving up music, television, sugar, or caffeine. Of course, I was going to take this assignment and mold it into another diet. I strived for perfection, and I thought giving up carbohydrates for six weeks and getting a perfect score would kill two birds with one stone. I imagined myself at the end of six weeks looking thinner, like something out of a diet commercial. People would admire my willpower, I thought.

The project, of course, did not go as planned. Part of the assignment was to journal throughout the process, and I found myself pouring my heart into the typed entries. I began to realize that my frustration was beyond what was typical for an assignment such as this. I hated my body. I hated food. I hated feeling deprived of something I desperately wanted. It was like a mirror had been held up, and I could finally see everything I had been doing to myself for the past 13 years. After three weeks, I gave up on the assignment but continued to journal my progress. I decided it was time to seek help.

I did not fully understand the extent of my problem, and it was difficult to decide where to turn first. Since I was part of an addictions course, I tried Overeaters Anonymous. After attending a few meetings, I decided that I needed a different kind of help. Like Goldilocks, I was searching for a fit that felt "just right." I decided to return to therapy, seeking out someone who specialized in eating disorders. I did not believe I had an eating disorder, at least not right away. I thought I had "issues with food," as I called it, but surely an eating disorders specialist could help me if she could help people with a problem like that.

Early on, I was diagnosed with BED. A discussion of my binge episodes, past history, and my relationship with food uncovered a problem that had been festering in my mind for more than a decade. On one hand, I was relieved to know that this was not a character flaw or a lack of willpower on my part, as the diet industry and my doctors would have me believe. All these years, I had been trying to cope with something millions of other people had also experienced. I was not alone. I was not an anomaly or a failure. I just needed help. Was I willing to accept it?

Recovery meant change in my life. The constant dieting had to stop, and it was difficult to give up in the beginning. On the one hand, there was this exhilarating freedom in knowing I could eat whatever I wanted. On the other hand, it was terrifying to realize that no one would tell me what I could and could not eat ever again. I had become used to certain rules: no carbohydrates for a month, no fruit for two weeks, no protein bigger than a deck of cards, no sugar, EVER. Without rules, who was I? What food was safe? At first, I stopped restricting but continued to binge, which resulted in weight gain. My mind told me that this was the proof that I could not live without some kind of restrictive diet. Yet I knew I did not have the heart to go back to starving myself again and pushed forward.

I continued to see a therapist and also began to work with a dietician, who started to teach me right away about paying attention to my hunger and full-ness signals. I had not realized that I had zero concept of what it was like to feel hunger and satiety without feeling the extremes of both. I did not know hunger without the rumbling stomach, the pain and dizziness that comes with not eating for long stretches of time. I did not know fullness without pain and becoming physically ill. When I realized that it was possible for me to feel full without overeating, and to eat enough that I would never be as hungry as I used to be, I was amazed. This helped me to stop bingeing and, therefore, stop gaining weight. It took a couple of years, but my weight stabilized.

Over the first two years of recovery, I saw an inordinate amount of change in my body, my spirit, and my mind. Food no longer held me prisoner. I could enjoy it and put it away when I was no longer hungry. I realized that food was not "good" or "bad," and that putting a moral value on food was keeping me stuck in my eating disorder. I began to exercise, and realized how strong I was and how great it felt to move my body. I would stumble and have a binge episode, or struggle with exercise, but I always went back to what I knew my body needed from me. Recovery became a part of my life and a number one priority. Yet there was one thing that kept me from getting the understanding and support of others, including medical professionals, friends, and family: I was still fat.

It seemed that people who knew me and knew about my recovery assumed I would lose weight as a result. When the pounds did not simply melt away,

I felt the pressure. If I was not bingeing but also not losing weight, then what *was* I doing? I felt the need to prove the value of my recovery to others, including my doctors. Often, doctors did not want to listen to my explanation of my eating disorder and my recovery. I would attempt to offer them a peek at my food journal, to have an open discussion about my exercise. I believed that because I was still fat, that meant I needed to justify that I was, indeed, healthy. I had to present evidence, because my body mass index said otherwise.

I would hope that a doctor would be willing to listen to his or her patients, especially when they make themselves vulnerable and share something like, "I've had an eating disorder since I was in the fourth grade and I am trying my hardest to get better." The sad truth is that research has proven otherwise. A 2013 study conducted by researchers at the Wake Forest School of Medicine found that 40 percent of medical students have a bias against fat patients and do not realize it.[4] Yet another 2013 study conducted at Johns Hopkins University School of Medicine concluded that their physicians did not build the same rapport and provide the same emotional support to fat patients as they did to patients of "normal" weight.[5]

In the Johns Hopkins study, researchers made recordings of doctors' interactions with 208 patients. While there was no difference in the amount of time spent with each patient, there was a discernible difference in the way the doctor spoke to overweight and obese patients. The study found that when speaking to those individuals, the doctors did not use nearly as many empathetic phrases as they did with "normal-weight" patients. When working with thinner patients, doctors showed more concern and reassured patients more frequently. The medical community is beginning to notice something I have experienced since I was a small child: fat people are not treated equally, and certainly not at the doctor's office.

I have experienced plenty of this type of judgment from physicians, and it did not end for me as a small child. Even after my diagnosis with BED, I have experienced discrimination on more than one occasion from various types of doctors. At first, I believed that explaining my situation to the doctor might help him or her understand the situation and therefore be more empathetic and informed. Sadly, this has not always been the case for me. I recall one doctor in particular who barely let me get the words "I'm seeing a dietician and a therapist" out of my mouth before he began to verbally abuse and berate me for my weight.

"You're going to die in ten years," he said to me. "You're going to get cirrhosis of your liver, and your skin is going to become jaundiced and turn yellow. Your eyes aren't going to be white anymore. It isn't cool, okay?"

"But, I . . . ," I stammered.

"How tall are you?" he demanded. I told him I was five foot four inches tall, at which point he told me I was supposed to weigh 110 pounds. Before I could even explain how unrealistic this was, he had another question.

"Does anyone in your family have diabetes?" he blurted. I told him yes, my grandfather had it toward the end of his life. Immediately, he launched into a tirade about how I would surely end up diabetic as well, even though my blood sugar had never been an issue in the past. All of his previous comments served as the foundation for his suggestion that I join a weight loss program being put on by the hospital. Which turned out to be not so much a suggestion as a demand, because he signed me up for that program without my consent.

That experience was the proverbial icing on the cake of all my horrendous doctor's appointments. I was traumatized by it, and afterward I experienced panic attacks simply from picking up the phone to call any doctor's office. I canceled appointments to avoid the humiliation and judgment that was surely forthcoming. It is a problem I am still struggling with and attempting to work through, for the sake of my physical well-being. I know that it is not a problem that is exclusive to me. Other people all over the world are experiencing the same thing each time they go to the doctor. There are people, like me, who are avoiding annual checkup appointments and necessary visits, simply as a way to shield themselves from the verbal abuse and humiliation that they experience from medical professionals.

Looking at the fact that medical professionals do have an antifat bias, and that they have been shown to be less empathetic and likely to bond with overweight and obese patients, it seems to be a reasonable conclusion that these physicians often lack the awareness and understanding to diagnose overweight and obese patients with an eating disorder. Think about it: if someone is already prejudiced against a person for her or his size, and does not try to emotionally connect and empathize with that person, how would that individual ever find out the person is struggling with an eating disorder?

Does fat prejudice keep physicians from asking the right questions in order to provide help to people with BED? Does that kind of environment make it more difficult for people to open up and tell their doctors what is really going on with their minds and bodies? I think about my own experiences, and it saddens me that not one doctor throughout the course of my life has asked me about my relationship with food. I try not to dwell on what could have been, but I cannot help but wish that at least one doctor had taken a moment to ask me a question, or express a concern that was not about the number on the scale but what was going on inside of me.

Perhaps this is lack of concern is why a Johns Hopkins School of Medicine study found that overweight and obese patients are more likely to switch doctors, or "doctor hop."[6] When one cannot find empathy or reassurance with a person whose job is to provide help, it is reasonable to assume that one will attempt to find better treatment elsewhere. What would be the point of continuing to spend time with a physician who cannot get past the size of your body?

Of course, physicians are not the only people with a bias toward fat people with eating disorders. That exists in society in general. One of the simplest examples is when I tell people I have an eating disorder, and they look at my body and say, *"Really?"* They sound incredulous, as if this could not possibly be. Yet I am obviously not the only fat person recovering from an eating disorder. I am a fat person with BED, the most common eating disorder out there. There are millions of people like me, and yet it is difficult not to feel alone. "Binge eating disorder" is not a term that simply tumbles from people's mouths in the way that "anorexia" or "bulimia" does.

I attended the National Eating Disorder Association's conference in 2012. I was thrilled to be present for many reasons, but mainly because I had looked over the agenda and seen at least two sessions devoted exclusively to discussing BED. It stunned me that professionals would be standing in front of a room full of people with a PowerPoint presentation talking about me. Well, not *me*, per se, but this disorder that had so deeply impacted my life and my body. Someone was going to get up and tell people that this was a real condition. To me, this meant that I was not a failure. I had not made a mistake. I experienced, and continue to experience, something very real and damaging, and I am not alone. For a professional to give credence to my experience, and that of millions of others, was an incredible gift.

The sessions on BED were very informative, and I was grateful to be a part of them. Yet those were only two of the many sessions I attended that weekend, and they were the only sessions on the subject. I noticed that during other sessions, BED did not come up at all or was mentioned only briefly, like an afterthought. I felt as though it was considered secondary to anorexia and bulimia throughout the course of the conference. It shocked me that even in the eating disorder community, there was still a bias. In my opinion, there seems to be a belief that people with eating disorders who are thin are going through something more severe or intense than those who are fat. Yes, when a person is severely underweight due to anorexia nervosa or bulimia nervosa, he or she may require more immediate medical attention, even hospitalization. Yet all eating disorders are severe, regardless of the body size of the person suffering from it.

It is prejudicial to believe that fat people do not suffer from eating disorders as much as thin people in the same circumstances. I deserve the same care at more than 200 pounds as a person half my size. My needs are equally as important. Yet this is not the experience I have had when dealing with medical professionals, the eating disorder community, and society in general. I feel as though I am being encouraged to continue engaging in eating disordered behaviors. Every diet commercial, every well-meaning friend or family member who discusses their newest restrictive food plan at length, every doctor who tells me to go on one fad diet or another, is contributing to the behaviors I fight every day to avoid.

Because I am fat, I am often asked in subtle ways to defend my recovery process. If a thin person wanted to give up dieting and practice intuitive eating, I doubt anyone would question it. But because of my size, many people have expressed surprise and concern that I would stop dieting, counting calories, and weighing myself. Why should I, *of all people*, decide it was okay to stop obsessing over my weight and the caloric value of each bite I put in my mouth? Nearly every day in a supermarket checkout lane, you can see magazines extolling thin people who have decided to be happy with their shape and stop obsessing over food. Where is the applause for the fat people who have decided to do the same and focus instead on their overall health and well-being?

We deserve better. It is unconscionable that fat people experience discrimination in every place that one should be able to find help and support. Body size should not be the factor that determines whether or not a person is treated with respect and dignity. That factor should be that we are all human, and we all deserve to be treated equally. It is a basic human right. We deserve doctors who listen, empathize, and are willing to be our partners in health, rather than our adversaries. For those of us who struggle with eating disorders, we deserve a community that recognizes our experiences and challenges as legitimate, one that wants to raise awareness and provide assistance to those of us who are struggling. We deserve to be uplifted and supported in our efforts to be well, physically, mentally, and spiritually.

As human beings, we are entitled to all of these things. Antifat bias is keeping us from receiving the support we all need. It will keep people from receiving the treatment and assistance they deserve, whether it is for an eating disorder or another medical condition. It will keep families from asking their loved ones the questions that could save their lives and help them find peace with their bodies. It is critical that we look beyond a person's size and see the person in front of us. Only then will we truly be a community that supports and assists people of all sizes.

NOTES

1. http://www.dsm5.org/documents/eating%20disorders%20fact%20sheet.pdf.

2. National Institute of Diabetes and Digestive and Kidney Diseases, "Binge Eating Disorder," last modified March 21, 2013, http://win.niddk.nih.gov/publications/binge.htm#foot3.

3. Binge Eating Disorder Association, "Characteristics," last modified June 2, 2013, http://bedaonline.com/understanding-bed/characteristics/.

4. Christopher Wanjek, "Obesity Bias Common among Medical Students," last modified May 28, 2013, http://www.livescience.com/34806-obesity-bias-medical-students-doctors.html?cmpid=514645.

5. Johns Hopkins Medicine, "Study: Physicians Less Likely to 'Bond' with Overweight Patients," last modified April 22, 2013, http://www.hopkinsmedicine.org/news/media/releases/study_physicians_less_likely_to_bond_with_overweight_patients.

6. Johns Hopkins Medicine, " 'Doctor Shopping' by Obese Patients Negatively Affects Health," last modified May 21, 2013, http://www.hopkinsmedicine.org/news/media/releases/doctor_shopping_by_obese_patients_negatively_affects_health

11

Exploring Weight Bias and Stigma: The Model of Appearance Perceptions and Stereotypes

Jennifer E. Copeland and Peter E. Jaberg

Are you a cheerleader? No, we are not asking if you have tried out for an organized cheering squad. Rather, in life, have you found yourself cheering others on to success or change? Oftentimes we are called upon as parents, partners, teachers, counselors, nurses, friends, to serve as an encouraging voice to others: "You can do it." "I am proud of you." "I knew you could." How often do you encounter someone who confides he or she is trying to lose weight, trying to get in shape for a vacation (with some reference to looking good in a swimsuit), or struggling with his or her latest dieting attempt? What do you say to such people? Is there awkwardness? Do you say nothing? Do you cheer them on?

Are you a judge? Again, the question is not whether you are an officer of the court. Rather, are you asked to judge: "Does this look good?" "Does this make me look fat?" Do you judge, whether asked or not? Do you play the role of polite magistrate who keeps lips sealed in the moment, exchanging polite social niceties—but passing harsh judgments in your thoughts, or perhaps making a judgmental comment to someone else after the person is out of earshot?

Are you a lonely person who finds it important to project confidence and power to others, but at the end of the day you have self-doubt and loathing? You know your feelings and thoughts might not be rational, but no matter how much success there is in life, you have looming doubts and perhaps downright hatred for your body or appearance. You know appearance shouldn't matter, but it does. Does anyone else know what this feels like?

The roles of cheerleader, judge, and lonely person are only three examples of ways we may relate to others (or ourselves) based on weight and appearance. Each of these is an understandable and functional role to adopt.

However, there are contexts in which each role is clearly inappropriate or less than optimal. The cheerleader role for weight loss is clearly inappropriate in the case of eating disorder, weight loss related to terminal disease, radical dieting behavior, or weight loss resulting from limb amputation. To illustrate this point imagine Lucile, a 72-year-old woman given such compliments several times over a three-month period: "You look wonderful; have you been losing weight?" "You have got to share your secret with me; you are losing weight and keeping it off." And, "Wow, you just keep losing weight—how skinny are you planning to get?" This last comment was the most telling. You see, Lucile had terminal cancer and did not want others to remember her as "a sick person." Why did everyone around her want to cheer her on to lose weight? She was not that large of a person to start. Ironically, had we known better we would have been cheering her to gain weight. What can be learned by reflecting on this story of cheerleading for Lucile?

The role of judge is one that is not always comfortable to admit. Some people outwardly and explicitly judge others for their weight and appearance. Others attempt to keep such judgments to themselves—or perhaps disclose them to others in private. Judgment is not inherently a bad thing. We make individual and social judgments every day as part of the decision-making process: Do I stop to get gas before I leave town or do I have enough to make it to work? Should I trust my child with this babysitter? Do we believe this candidate will serve the public interest? Judging others for their appearance, weight, or apparent health can, at times, seem a logical progression of these thoughts and actions.

We are constantly bombarded with media messages that obesity is bad and overweight is a national (U.S.) epidemic to be fought against. "Shouldn't a fat person do more to become healthy and fit? Wouldn't they be so much happier?" Assumptions about individuals who are skinny should be similarly questioned: "Wow, you must have great control!" "She must be uptight." "I wonder if she ever throws up on purpose?" And, "are you from Africa?"— (this statement being an insensitive reference to starvation from famine found in some areas of the African continent). Even if we think we are adequately hiding our thoughts, oftentimes our nonverbal behaviors communicate hurtful judgment. Sometimes, we are heard when we don't realize it. Sometimes, the assumptions we hold inside hurt others whether we intend them to or not.

Perhaps most importantly, the judgments (assumptions and biases) we hold about weight, appearance, and health can hurt ourselves as much as, if not more than, they can hurt others. What are your assumptions about your weight, appearance, and health? There are the truths we are comfortable and proud to admit to ourselves—and there may be truths inside our being more painful to acknowledge. Yet our biases can hurt ourselves and others in very concrete ways. How then might a person think about and change weight bias?

It is in the interest of aiding you to consider and explore your own biases and assumptions related to appearance, weight, and health that we share this chapter with you. How do one's assumptions and beliefs change over time? How does learning impact one's assumptions related to weight? If you can identify with one of these roles (i.e., cheerleader, judge, lonely person), what does that mean for you and what comes next? In reflecting on these questions, we were led to develop a model for weight bias. More specifically, how might a variety of people experience thoughts, behaviors, emotions related to weight and weight bias (toward self and others)?

The Model of Appearance Perceptions and Stereotypes (MAPS) was developed based upon the integration of qualitative data, examination of relevant literature, and the worldviews of the authors. It serves as a framework for assessing level of weight-based discrimination regarding personal weight and the weight of others or, conversely, the degree of acceptance of body size and weight. This model was developed to increase social dialogue surrounding weight bias and ultimately serve as a tool to facilitate the acceptance of size diversity. Initially, we labeled this model "F.A.T.S.O." (Fat Acceptance Towards Self and Others). In addition to being descriptive of the model, the acronym was meant to serve as a provocative moniker to get the reader emotionally activated. We intended that some readers might be offended, others would laugh or snicker, and yet others would appreciate the play on words. It was our intent to get the reader thinking about his or her assumptions and biases from the beginning. Perhaps our approach was too effective. We received feedback that our acronym was too controversial or too arousing, suggesting a more neutral title would be more appropriate. We discussed what this feedback might mean, if changing the name would be appropriate or whether it would represent an unnecessary or potentially inappropriate concession to others' biases. Even as we write this, we have lingering doubts as to whether or not we made the right decision.

The MAPS framework was based in part upon the interpretation of qualitative data; the data were examined for "patterned response or meaning"[1] at multiple levels utilizing thematic analysis.[2] Additional analysis with a grounded theory approach[3] yielded distinct stages regarding subjective perceptions of "obesity," related mental health experiences, and the degree of personal control over weight. A description of MAPS and its stages was shared with subject matter experts in the areas of size diversity, weight bias, and health for further feedback and analysis, which was considered and integrated into the model as appropriate. Challenges included recognition of the intersection of other elements of diversity, the role of healthism, and potential bias perpetuated via the language of the model.

The MAPS model is intended to evoke a process of both reflection and introspection. It is described in terms of an individual's thoughts, behaviors, emotions, level of education and/or knowledge, and self-perceptions. The model is not exclusively linear or systemic in nature. One may progress as well as regress through the stages due to personal experiences, education or training, or interactions with individuals of different body weights and sizes. The direction of one's development would likely occur from one stage to the next without skipping a step. Each of the stages is not meant to be discrete, and overlap may be present among the elements within and between the stages.

We do not share this developmental model with you from on high as often happens in education. Rather, we respectfully approach the topic and the model from a position of humility. As we started our journey studying weight bias, we found we were learning as much about ourselves as those we studied. We were forced to confront our own assumptions and biases. We began a path of confronting positive and affirming, as well as destructive and potentially hurtful, beliefs and assumptions. We had to confront each other about the language we used, how we talked, and how we related to each other. Consistent with the model we describe, we are not there yet on our own journeys. The highest level of development is an ideal, an aspiration to chase, but perhaps never quite reach. We are all human and must be realistic about our relatively short time on the planet.

We recognize the considerable influence of our own narratives on the development of the MAPS model. Many choices for the content and structure of this model were influenced by our growth and development. Our world-views were influenced not only by personal experiences but also by engagement with relevant literature and advanced training, as well as changed interactions with marginalized populations. One of us grew up with fat friends and family. While internally adhering to biased attitudes, she experienced discomfort with the resulting harm to others. It was not until being exposed to research and alternative viewpoints during graduate-level training that she fully appreciated the consequences of weight bias and began working to improve her own awareness and understanding. The other author grew up with the benefits of privilege (i.e., size, gender, and race/ethnicity). Now familiar with concepts such as body image and body effectiveness, it is grieving to witness the psychological torment of weight bias. He cherishes the opportunity to challenge himself and others to reflect on weight assumptions and behaviors. It is through the lens of these worldviews that data were examined, literature evaluated, and the model formed.

Recognizing this humanity, as you read about the model and consider your own thoughts, beliefs, and behaviors, the point is not to assume you are in any particular stage or level, but rather to reflect on what aspects of each stage may or may not fit you. The remainder of the chapter is dedicated to presenting options for continued growth and development in your own weight bias journey. It is unlikely to be quick or easy, but take solace in this: your awareness of and willingness to consider the need for growth will be your greatest strengths in this journey.

BLATANT WEIGHTISM (LEVEL 1)

The first level is marked by overt or blatant discrimination based on perceived weight status (see Table 11.1 for a summary). A high degree of blame or responsibility is placed on the individual for his or her weight status. No acceptance of the weight of one's self or others is present. Rather, weight- and appearance-related thoughts, behaviors, and attitudes are revered in a derogatory manner.

TABLE 11.1   Level 1: Blatant Weightism

Thoughts:	Characterized by stereotypes and adherence to cultural ideals of weight, health, and beauty. Weight is linked with value and worth (i.e., self and others). Weight status is due to the assumed lack of appropriate diet and exercise.
Behaviors:	Overt antifat statements and actions that might result in discrimination. Interpersonal relationships might be altered or restricted based on an individual's weight status.
Emotions:	Experience disgust or strong dislike when encountering individuals perceived to be "overweight." Experience shame for relationships or associations with individuals who are perceived to be "overweight."
Education:	Little to no education in weight-related issues. Knowledge consists of social stereotypes and commonly accepted myths related to weight and health.
Self:	Unlikely to claim weight as an element of their self. Likely to hold themselves to the thin ideal of beauty as they would others.

Being fat is thought to be the direct result of a perceived lack of appropriate health-related choices and behaviors. There may be an assumption of individual fault or responsibility for weight and appearance (i.e., an individual made the choice to be this way—it is his or her fault). Weight and appearance are strongly linked such that individuals who are perceived to be fat are thought to be of little value. Individuals perceived to be fat are thought to be morally weak (i.e., lacking in the willpower, discipline, fortitude, desire, etc., to achieve and maintain a "healthy" weight). Underlying each stereotype is an acceptance and internalization of the thin ideal of beauty, or the idea that only individuals perceived to be "thin" are attractive.

EMERGING AWARENESS (LEVEL 2)

Individuals at this level of development are differentiated from those at Level 1 development by the integration of additional information regarding

TABLE 11.2 Level 2: Emerging Awareness

Thoughts:	Weight status is the result of biological determinants (e.g., genetics, diet, exercise). Adherence to cultural ideals of beauty. Recognition of the existence of weight-based stigmatization and bias present in society.
Behaviors:	Covert antifat statements and actions in public contexts that might result in discrimination. Behaviors are comparatively less aggressive and severe than Level 1. Explicit behaviors are prevalent in private situations.
Emotions:	Experience pity for individuals perceived to be "overweight." Uncomfortable with perceived "overweight" in self and others. Worry about the health status of those they are intimately acquainted with who are perceived to be "overweight," but do not act on these concerns.
Education:	Have acquired some knowledge beyond that of basic social stereotypes and myths.
Self:	If they see their self as "overweight," they might struggle with this, seeing it as their 'fault." Weight is linked to personal worth and value. Do not see this as weight bias.

weight and health into one's perspective (see Table 11.2 for a summary). A person is less rigid about explanations of weight, health, and its development. A decrease in the severity of discriminatory thoughts and behaviors of Level 1 is likely to be observed. Moderate to high blame or fault is placed on an individual for his or her perceived weight status. Yet there still is no acceptance of the weight or size of the self or others.

Individuals likely place a strong emphasis on the diet and exercise behaviors of self and others. They may seek to hold themselves and others to a strict dietary regimen in order to prevent an "unhealthy" weight. Explicit statements and behaviors are likely to be more prevalent in private situations as compared to public environments, such as the bullying or pressuring of family members perceived to be "obese" about their weight and health. Discrimination against fat individuals may be present, particularly if exposure to divergent views or disapproving feedback has not occurred.

BENEVOLENT WEIGHTISM (LEVEL 3)

Increasing awareness about weight, health, and weight-related stigmatization, as well as a willingness to act on these issues, characterizes benevolent weightism (see Table 11.3 for a summary). Low to moderate blame is placed on an individual for his or her perceived weight status. There is low to moderate acceptance of the weight status of a fat person.

Although the individual questions the standard of care (i.e., traditional ideas regarding weight and health, fat and weight loss, etc.[4]), he or she continues to conceptualize weight as something to be managed or controlled.

TABLE 11.3   Level 3: Benevolent Weightism

Thoughts:	Realization of the discrepancies within the "obesity" argument, which might be accompanied by distress. Questions the claims of the status quo perceptions. Adherence to cultural ideals of beauty.
Behaviors:	Characterized by the cheerleader role. Do not seek to explicitly discriminate against individuals perceived as "overweight." Make extraordinary efforts to "help."
Emotions:	Growing empathy for those perceived as "overweight." Experience of frustration or distress because of attempts to reconcile internal cognitive dissonance.
Education:	Knowledge base beyond social stereotypes from formal or informal education. Have been exposed to information about weight, health, appearance, and discrimination.
Self:	More accepting of the weight of others than their own. Might be conscious of personal biases but might not be willing to consciously admit this.

They are unlikely to be familiar with the potential harm associated with weight loss interventions.[5] The "cheerleader role" is undertaken with the goal of inspiring others to finally make the necessary changes to lose weight. Individuals at this level may make efforts to "bend over backwards" to "help" individuals who are fat. Although this may be viewed as condescending by some, the individual in this stage of development is likely to feel self-assured regarding his or her benevolence. That is, the individual believes he or she is doing the "right thing."

QUESTIONING THE STATUS QUO (LEVEL 4)

People in the fourth level challenge their personal beliefs about appearance and weight status quo after becoming disillusioned with the commonly accepted ideas of fat (see Table 11.4 for a summary). Low to no blame is assigned for weight status. There is moderate acceptance of the weight status of self and others.

The hallmark of Level 4 is cognitive dissonance, such that adherence to one set of beliefs may be logically opposed to another set of beliefs as the individual attempts to reconcile the contradictions. An internal realization of opposing traditional weight and health knowledge has occurred and may be associated with some form of distress. The individual is debating such issues as: the status quo understanding of fat versus alternative ideas of weight and health; personal responsibility for weight status versus the inclusion of social, institutional, and/or governmental influences on health and weight; and biological determinants of weight versus individual behavior and/or lifestyle factors. Although adherence to the idea of personal responsibility for weight

TABLE 11.4   Level 4: Questioning the Status Quo

Thoughts:	Characterized by uncertainty regarding the status quo understanding of weight, health, and beauty. Weight/size is not fully accepted and is conceptualized as a thing to fight against.
Behaviors:	Advocate for individuals perceived to be "overweight," including decreasing weight-based discrimination, in self and others.
Emotions:	Anger/frustration due to the observation of the poor treatment of individuals perceived to be "overweight."
Education:	Knowledge base includes information of the extent of weight bias in society, the role of social/cultural factors in weight and health.
Self:	Contradictions exist between beliefs for self and beliefs for others. Continue to be more accepting of the weight of others than self. Attempt to integrate disparate beliefs into more coherent understanding.

is present, an emphasis is placed upon poor choices in the context of a toxic or obesogenic environment. The thin ideal of beauty is used as the standard for themselves and others but is reflectively questioned.

EMBRACING CONTRADICTIONS (LEVEL 5)

A release of adherence to the commonly accepted approaches to weight and health is the hallmark of this level (see Table 11.5 for a summary). The perception of individual blame and personal responsibility for weight is minimized. There is moderate to high acceptance of the weight status of self and others. The fifth level represents the highest level of development observed in the data.

The individual no longer holds opinions consistent with the standard of care related to weight and health, wherein recognition of the multitude of factors that contribute to weight status has occurred. An awareness of weight bias and thin privilege exists, as well as the corresponding impact on physiological and psychological health. Their actions are characterized by a diminished focus on weight loss or the pursuit of a goal weight. Instead, individuals will likely direct their effort toward well-being, health, and/or health behaviors for those who desire it and may incorporate the Health at Every Size principles.[6] The remaining implicit beliefs held by self and others are explicitly challenged such that the individual may attempt to persuade individuals of a lower level of development to become more enlightened.

The ideal level of weight acceptance, as conceptualized by imperfect individuals, is characterized by a full integration of thoughts, behaviors, and emotions into one's experience of self and others. There is no judgment of self or others' weight status. The individual is aware of weight bias, thin privilege,

TABLE 11.5   Level 5: Embracing Contradictions

Thoughts:	Have achieved an understanding of the multifactorial nature of weight and health. Decreased adherence to cultural ideals of weight, health, and beauty. Meaningfully consider the influence of weight bias and thin privilege. Are aware of a connection between weight bias and eating disorders.
Behaviors:	Advocate for individuals perceived to be "overweight," including making efforts to influence others related to these beliefs and the social injustice of weight bias. Challenge perceptions (e.g., personal, professional) of beauty and weight.
Emotions:	Discomfort associated with discussions of weight loss, dieting, and so forth, without shared beliefs or enlightenment.
Education:	Knowledge base includes information related to the alternative means of improving health, the ineffectiveness of diet and weight loss in improving health, the complexity of factors in weight and health, a relationship between weight bias and eating disorders.
Self:	Increased acceptance of personal weight and health status. Successful but incomplete integration of ideas related to weight, health, and beauty.

and the associated power dynamics. Personal perceptions of weight and appearance hold no influence over interpersonal or social judgments of value, worth, respect, or humanity.

There is recognition of the multitude of factors that may influence weight and health status. The relationship between weight bias and eating disorders is acknowledged and accounted for in related interventions. Overall well-being and healthy lifestyle is advocated for individuals who desire it, and improvements are seen as beneficial for all individuals regardless of their size, weight, and health status. The individual would experience and display compassion and patience toward individuals of a lower level of weight acceptance. In this manner the individual may work to help others grow and mature toward the same ideal state.

CHARTING A DIFFERENT COURSE

Weight-based discrimination is among the most pervasive biases in modern society. Each of us has internalized these attitudes in ways that uniquely affect our lives. Our responses are influenced by a multitude of factors including family environments, peers, and even our own weight status. Side effects of weight bias are not limited to those who are the overt targets. Rather, those who are thin face bias as well.[7]

Each of us has assumptions and biases related to weight, appearance, and health to explore. For some this may necessitate the guidance of a qualified mental health professional in order to explore and challenge long-standing hostility. Others should enlist the assistance of a trusted individual to provide feedback about the things said and done that may harm others. What is universally important is to continue challenging yourself to grow. Do not expect radical change to happen overnight. It took years to develop our thoughts and attitudes, and it will take time to undo them. Spend time with people you admire and who inspire you; these positive institutions and positive environments are vital for providing support, encouragement, and feedback for change. The key is willingness to be honest and open, and to maintain humility to admit wrongdoing as necessary.

Achieving increasing freedom from the confines of bias and privilege next requires affirming your intentions. Contemplate what you would like to practice and see transformed in your life. Establish a vision for the growth you would like to see happen. Begin by determining your starting point via such tools as the Implicit Association Test,[8] which assess attitudes of which you may not be readily aware. Then commit to becoming more mindful of your thoughts. Pay attention to what comes to mind about weight and health throughout the day. Track these (in a journal, in a notebook, or on your smartphone) to help you identify triggers, patterns, and specific areas for improvement. Is your level of knowledge and understanding keeping you from considering other viewpoints? For professionals, address this by submersing yourself in the research and scientific journals such as *Fat Studies: An Interdisciplinary Journal of Body Weight and Society* or engaging with professional organizations such as the Association for Size Diversity and Acceptance or the National Association to Advance Fat Acceptance. For nonprofessionals, find resources that break down important data for people at all levels of scientific understanding. Consider reviewing Linda Bacon's *Health at Every Size: The Surprising Truth about Your Weight;*[9] Paul Campos's *The Obesity Myth: Why America's Obsession with Weight Is Hazardous to Your Health;*[10] Glenn Gaesser's *Big Fat Lies: The Truth about Your Weight and Health;*[11] and/or J. Eric Oliver's *Fat Politics: The Real Story Behind America's Obesity Epidemic.*[12]

When faced with bias it's quite easy to feel enraged, hopeless, and even defeated. Those who have been subject to this know firsthand the hurt that follows including increased depression and anxiety,[13] higher incidence of binge eating behaviors,[14] more body dissatisfaction,[15] and less desirable health behaviors.[16] Emotional reactions are normal, especially considering all that society has trained us to do. It is important to honor the experiences that lead one to hold these thoughts, behave in this way, dislike others based on their size or weight, and likely to inflict these same things on oneself. For those who are confronted with this bias in daily life, the strongest weapon is not a weapon; it is, in fact, compassion that can be most powerful. Aggressively challenging individuals exhibiting deeply ingrained beliefs is likely to only set them on the defensive, holding on all the more strongly to their perceptions. Instead, gentle challenging and exposure to new viewpoints will be the most helpful. Research in multiple areas of culture and diversity has indicated that activities exposing one to novel situations and the minority group, developing empathy, and taking perspective are important in altering attitudes and perceptions.[17] Share the newest literature debunking contemporary understandings of weight and health. Assertively stating when your feelings are hurt by others' actions may be even more important, helping to connect that individual's behaviors with the logical consequences—hurting others.

Change happens not only in our perceptions but also within our actions. Practice self-compassion, honoring feelings of guilt that arise as you develop more awareness. Do not linger on these or allow them to hijack your world. True healing comes with each moment and opportunity we have to practice compassion with others as well as ourselves. That weight bias has wreaked havoc and brought pain for many in this world is not questioned. Research has clearly documented the impact on health and well-being.[18] Anger and resentments toward those who may have inflicted that harm are barriers to lasting change. Cultivate loving kindness for these individuals as well as ourselves, modeling the possibilities we hope will come to fruition. As Thich Nhat Hanh[19] encouraged: "Only dwelling in the present can make us free. We have to look into our suffering, our craving. And when we see its face we will smile: you cannot make me your prisoner any more."

NOTES

1. Virginia Braun and Victoria Clarke, "Using Thematic Analysis in Psychology," *Qualitative Research in Psychology* 3, no. 2 (2006): 82.

2. Richard E. Boyatzis, *Transforming Qualitative Information: Thematic Analysis and Code Development* (Thousand Oaks, CA: Sage, 1998); Braun and Clarke, "Using Thematic Analysis," 77–101.

3. Karen Henwood and Nick Pidgeon, "Grounded Theory in Psychological Research," in *Qualitative Research in Psychology: Expanding Perspectives in Methodology and Design*, ed. Paul M. Camice et al. (Washington, DC: American Psychological Association, 2003), 131–55.

4. National Institutes of Health, *Clinical Guidelines on the Identification, Evaluation, and Treatment of Overweight and Obesity in Adults: The Evidence Report* (Washington, DC: U.S. Government Printing Office, 1998).

5. Michelle Laliberte et al., "Controlling Your Weight versus Controlling Your Lifestyle: How Beliefs about Weight Control Affect Risk for Disordered Eating, Body Dissatisfaction, and Self-Esteem," *Cognitive Therapy and Research* 31, no. 6 (2007): 853–69; Dianne Neumark-Sztainer et al., "Obesity, Disordered Eating, and Eating Disorders in a Longitudinal Study of Adolescents: How Do Dieters Fare 5 Years Later?," *Journal of the American Dietetic Association* 106, no. 4 (2006): 559–68; Jane

Ogden and Catherine Whyman, "The Effect of Repeated Weighing on Psychological State," *European Eating Disorders Review* 5, no. 2 (1997): 121–30.

6. Association for Size Diversity and Health, "Health at Every Size® Principles," accessed February 5, 2013, https://www.sizediversityandhealth.org/content.asp?id=152; Deborah Burgard, "Developing Body Trust: A Body-Positive Approach to Treating Eating Disorders," in *Effective Clinical Practice in the Treatment of Eating Disorders: The Heart of the Matter*, ed. Margo Maine et al. (New York: Routledge, 2009); Karin Kratina, "Health at Every Size: Clinical Applications," *Healthy Weight Journal* 17, no. 2 (2003): 19–23; Jon Robison, "Health at Every Size: Antidote for the 'Obesity Epidemic,' " *Healthy Weight Journal* 17, no. 1 (January 2003): 4–7.

7. Viren Swami et al., "An Investigation of Weight Bias against Women and Its Associations with Individual Difference Factors," *Body Image* 7, no. 3 (2010): 194–99; Kristy Zwickert and Elizabeth Rieger, "Stigmatizing Attitudes towards Individuals with Anorexia Nervosa: An Investigation of Attribution Theory," *Journal of Eating Disorders* 1 (2013), accessed February 5, 2013, doi:10.1186/2050-2974-1-5.

8. "Project Implicit," accessed May 1, 2013, http://implicit.harvard.edu.

9. Linda Bacon, *Health at Every Size: The Surprising Truth about Your Weight* (Dallas, TX: BenBella Books, 2008).

10. Paul Campos, *The Diet Myth: Why America's Obsession with Weight Is Hazardous to Your Health* (New York: Penguin, 2004).

11. Glenn Gaesser, *Big Fat Lies: The Truth about Your Weight and Health* (Carlsbad, CA: Gürze Books, 2002).

12. J. Eric Oliver, *Fat Politics: The Real Story Behind America's Obesity Epidemic* (Oxford: Oxford University Press, 2006).

13. Laura E. Durso and Janet D. Latner, "Understanding Self-Directed Stigma: Development of the Weight Bias Internalization Scale," *Obesity* 16, no. S2 (2008): S80–S86.

14. Robert A. Carels et al., "Implicit, Explicit, and Internalized Weight Bias and Psychosocial Maladjustment among Treatment-Seeking Adults," *Eating Behaviors* 11 (2010): 180–85.

15. Lenny R. Vartanian and Jacqueline G. Shaprow, "Effects of Weight Stigma on Exercise Motivation and Behavior: A Preliminary Investigation among College-Aged Females," *Journal of Health Psychology* 13 (2008): 131–38.

16. Robert A. Carels et al., "Weight Bias and Weight Loss Treatment Outcomes in Treatment-Seeking Adults," *Annals of Behavioral Medicine* 37 (2009): 350–55.

17. Diana Burgess et al., "Reducing Racial Bias among Health Care Providers: Lessons from Social-Cognitive Psychology," *Society of General Internal Medicine* 22 (2007): 882–997; Sigrún Daníelsdóttir, Kerry S. O'Brien, and Anna Ciao, "Anti-Fat Prejudice Reduction: A Review of Published Studies," *Obesity Facts* 3 (2010): 47–58; Krystina A. Finlay and Walter G. Stephan, "Improving Intergroup Relations: The Effects of Empathy on Racial Attitudes," *Journal of Applied Social Psychology* 30, no. 8 (2000): 1720–37; Adam D. Galinsky and Gordon B. Moskowitz, "Perspective Taking: Decreasing Stereotype Expression, Stereotype Accessibility, and In-Group Favoritism," *Journal of Personality and Social Psychology* 78, no. 4 (2000): 708–24; Thomas F. Pettigrew, "Intergroup Contact Theory," *Annual Review of Psychology* 49

(1998): 65–85; Xiangyu Zuo and Shihui Han, "Cultural Experiences Reduce Racial Bias in Neural Responses to Others' Suffering," *Culture and Brain* 1, no. 1 (2013): 34–46.

18. Janet Latner, Laura Durso, and Jonathan Mond, "Health and Health-Related Quality of Life among Treatment-Seeking Overweight and Obese Adults: Associations with Internalized Weight Bias," *Journal of Eating Disorders* 1 (2013), accessed February 5, 2013, doi:10.1186/2050-2974-1-3.

19. "On Meditation," *Shambhala Sun*, March 2003, accessed May 1, 2013, http://www.shambhalasun.com/index.php?option=com_content&task=view&id=2908&Itemid=0.

12

Working with Eating Disorders and Body Image Using Expressive Arts Therapies

Deah Schwartz

The size of someone's body is not an indicator of eating disorders or issues with body image or body dissatisfaction. People of all sizes experience these conditions, but as a therapist specializing with this population, I think it's important to look at our society's obsession with a stereotype of beauty as a common contributor to these issues in people of size, and to look at what we can do to best help people who are the victims. In that vein I think that working to help people change their relationships with their bodies—rather than suggesting that they should change their bodies as a way to escape social stigma—is a form of activism.

Expressive arts therapies, also known as therapeutic arts or creative arts therapy, is a multimodality approach to treating a wide array of diagnoses. The creative arts therapist engages the client/patient in sessions that employ art, music, movement, drama, filmmaking, storytelling, or writing, in order to facilitate healing, improve quality of life, and address treatment goals and objectives in the cognitive, social, emotional, and physical domains. But let's take a quick look at why expressive arts therapy is an exceptionally good fit for treating people struggling with eating disorders, body dissatisfaction, and body image.

TIME IS *NOT* ON OUR SIDE

In a perfect world we would have as much time as a client needed to work therapeutically. Unfortunately, in these days of managed care and economic hardship, time is an intervening variable that cannot be ignored. The value of using therapeutic arts as a treatment intervention is based on many premises, one of which is that the creative process involved in the act of artistic expression can more *efficiently* tap into a person's ability to access information that is elusive and resistant to traditional verbal psychotherapy or cognitive behavioral approaches.[1] People struggling with eating disorders and body dysmorphia (distorted body image) are typically very bright, verbal, *and* feel detached from their body. It is not uncommon to hear clients make statements such as "I hate my body," or "I would be fine if my body would just change." There is the person and there is "that body." From their perspective, the body is not part of the person, it is a separate entity. The more they talk in a session, the more the split between their mind and body is evidenced. When one of the goals of therapy is to integrate mind and body, overintellectualizing and excessive verbal processing in a session can be contraindicated and make this objective more difficult to attain. I often reference this as a *talking head*: the disassociation from the body so profound that for all intents and purposes their bodies could be in another room as we explore their self-hate, food obsessions, and feelings of hopelessness just on the other side of the wall. When our sessions remain purely verbal, the client tends to talk in loops, replicating the cyclical nature of his or her eating disorder and weight-cycling patterns. At the end of the session, little if any integration may have been accomplished and noticeable progress is difficult to assess. Conversely, when I incorporate expressive arts and recreational therapies in sessions, it is an entirely different story. We are able to access salient information more quickly and work on tangible coping strategies to achieve a more positive and integrated sense of self.

NO RIGHT OR WRONG

The quest for perfection and feeling in control is an additional factor shared by people with an eating disorder or body dissatisfaction.[2] Living up to an ideal of perfection, trying to please others, and judging oneself primarily based on physical appearance are persistent driving forces that lead to body hate and disordered eating.[3] Because the primary focus of therapeutic arts is on the *process* of creation and not the final product, the clients learn how to appreciate who they are in the moment, explore reasons for their behaviors, and establish new barometers for self-acceptance. From day one in my sessions I explain to clients that in expressive arts therapies, there is no right or wrong in what they create. They are not a writer, actress, painter, or dancer—they are writing, acting, painting, and dancing. No one is judging them based on any standardized measure of talent, beauty, or success. In fact, this is a safe place where there is respect and admiration for individuality, and each person is given permission to explore qualities that make him or her unique.

VARIETY IS THE SPICE OF LIFE

Expressive arts therapists are trained to use a variety of modalities and employ them either separately or together in sessions. Why use a multimodality approach? When Howard Gardner first came out with his book *Frames of Intelligence: The Theory of Multiple Intelligences*,[4] many teachers and behavioral health practitioners embraced the concept. After all, if people are not wired to learn or process information in the same way, why not offer a menu of options? Taking that a step further, why would we expect people to resonate with the same form of art expression? How wonderful for a client to be able to access therapeutic information and address treatment issues using the modality that most suits her or him. When a therapist is able to move from modality to modality based on a person's comfort level and interest, there are more opportunities to facilitate expression and insight.

The level of perceived risk is another factor. Some modalities are less threatening than others. A writing exercise may be less frightening than a theater directive at first for those who feel uncomfortable with people looking at their body. Others may resonate with or feel safer doing collage work instead of dance. Film and video are also powerful modalities. When a person watches someone else talking about or depicting similar issues with eating disorders or body image issues, it makes it easier to follow suit. When I show clips from the DVD of the theater piece *Leftovers, the Ups and Downs of a Compulsive Eater*,[5] where three women disclose their inner secrets about their body shame, disordered eating behaviors, deep despair, and desperate attempts to lose weight in order to be accepted into their peer group, family, and/or society, clients often feel safe enough to share more of their personal story about food and body image. It is akin to priming a pump or giving a battery a jump start. If someone else is disclosing, then there is tacit permission to do the same.

THE POWER OF METAPHOR

All of the expressive arts modalities allow the client and therapist to work with metaphors, and metaphors are powerful back doors, side doors, trap doors into material that may have been locked away in nooks and crannies, masking triggers and impeding progress. Some symbols that are used or generated via expressive arts directives are archetypal, which provides a common ground for building mutual understanding between the therapist and the client. Other symbols are more personal and subjective; hence they can activate thoughts, feelings, and *aha moments* that resemble a reflex action bypassing the censoring of the more linear left brain process. For example, imagine you are exploring the reasons why a client chooses body hate over body acceptance. What are their fears or assumptions about choosing to accept themselves in lieu of perpetuating their belief that the only way to be "good" is to lose weight and be thinner? What will they gain? What will they lose? What will change? What will stay the same? Frequently, if these questions are asked directly, many clients will have a difficult time answering or their answers may be superficial or parroting the messages that have been fed to them over the years. An expressive arts therapist may instead put out a pile of keys and say, "Choose one key that opens the door to body acceptance and one key that opens the door to body hate. Now choosing from the art materials provided, create a drawing, painting, or collage that shows what is behind each of those doors."

The visual cue and metaphor of the key unlocks the creative process, which often taps into a deeper subconscious awareness that may be missed when merely answering a direct question. In addition, the finished piece of artwork is a tangible outcome of the information harvested during the session that can be used in future sessions to work deeper on the material generated. Movement, dance, and theater also provide fertile ground for exploring issues that pertain to body hate by using the body as part of the therapeutic process. Once a "safe container" (a therapeutic space where the client knows he or she is safe) is established for clients where they are certain they are not there to prove they are a worthy contestant for *Dancing with the Stars*, they are free to find ways to use *their body* to express feelings about *their body*. This is one of the earliest steps in declaring a truce in the war between their self-esteem and their body. With the critical mind removed from the equation, a deeper appreciation for what their body *can* do and what ability they already have can be generated. Practicing new behaviors is more than just a cognitive behavioral exercise in practicing new responses to emotional triggers; it can be imperative to use the body itself to practice new behaviors and try on new ways of moving in the world. If one learns to love and live in one's body in the here and now, the way one moves one's body will change. The self-esteem that grows from cultivating self-love and self-acceptance will generalize into other areas of life.

When I was the director of the Expressive Arts Therapy Department at a psychiatric hospital in the Bay Area, there were many ways we categorized our patients. One way was to separate the voluntary admissions from the involuntary admissions. The label "voluntary admit" came with an assumption that this patient was ready to change. Conversely, it was widely believed that those who were "involuntary admits" were being forced to change. In both cases, change was a treatment goal. In both cases, resistance was a formidable barrier to actualizing change. Even the voluntary patients with the internal desire to change bumped up against the walls of resistance.

When people embark on the road to size acceptance, which may or may not include changing their ways of eating or their relationship with food, it is often as a result of negative results from a long history of external pressure to be different from what they are. They have been told over and over to change. "Change your diet. Change your body. Change your behavior. Change your appearance." The overriding message is, "You are not okay."

When we hear these messages over and over, they become internalized and we develop ways to try to make ourselves okay, some of which include self-destructive and self-mutilating behaviors. Changing the way we feel about ourselves, loving ourselves as we are, is rarely presented as an option.

I worked with a young woman who told me, "If I ever kill myself, tell people it was because I couldn't stand facing another day looking in the mirror and starting the day off hating myself." She felt like a failure, every morning, because she couldn't change herself in the way that others wanted her to change. The only definition of change she could articulate or imagine was to change the way she looked to please her family.

Using art, drama, and movement, we worked on redefining her criteria for change. We looked at why others had the authority to create *her* change menu. We looked at what she would change about herself if no one else had a say and she could just change what she wanted. We explored her resistance to change, inside and out.

One day in our drama therapy group she announced that she was doing a scene about the two things she wanted to change about herself more than anything. The group waited. Would it be her butt? Her thighs? Her upper arms?

Her scene was enthralling, powerful, humorous, and poignant. It incorporated many of the metaphors and symbols she had discovered and used in her writing and artwork over the past three weeks working in my group. As the scene ended, she was in a restaurant. She ordered her selections from *The Change Menu*:

> For my main course, I'll have the not giving my power of self-acceptance away to my family. And for dessert, I'll have the learning to speak Spanish fluently please.

It's been a while since I heard from this patient, but from time to time I like to think of her sitting in a restaurant, perhaps in Barcelona, speaking perfect Spanish and loving herself as she is.

Keeping the metaphor of a menu in mind and the variety of options most menus offer, the elements that contribute to a person developing an eating disorder or body dissatisfaction are numerous and complex. They include genetic predisposition, environmental factors, cultural paradigms, and familial role models. It is my experience that a multifaceted diagnosis benefits from a multimodality approach. Please, let me emphasize that I am *not* saying that verbal psychotherapy, cognitive behavioral, or dialectical behavioral therapies are ineffective in treating eating disorders and body image issues. What I am saying is that an expressive arts therapeutic approach is an additional efficacious intervention for facilitating change and healing that integrates the whole person—body, mind, and spirit.

NOTES

1. D. Weiner, *Beyond Talk Therapy: Using Movement and Expressive Techniques in Clinical Practice* (Washington, DC: American Psychological Association, 1999).

2. P. L. Hewett, G. L. Fiett, and E. Ediger, "Perfectionism Traits and Perfectionistic Self-Presentation in Eating Disorder Attitudes, Characteristics, and Symptoms," *International Journal of Eating Disorders* 18, no. 4 (1995): 317–26.

3. P. Campos, *The Diet Myth: Why America's Obsession with Weight Is Hazardous to Your Health* (New York: Penguin, 2004).

4. Howard Gardner, *Frames of Intelligence: The Theory of Multiple Intelligences* (New York: Basic Books, 1983).

5. D. Schwartz and A. Wilford, *Leftovers* workbook/DVD set (Oakland, CA: ETTA, 2008).

13

A "Weigh" to Go? Looking at School-Based Antifat Interventions from a Weight-Based versus a Health-Based Approach

Dr. Ameerah Mattar

The issue of childhood obesity has, undoubtedly, been depicted as a serious public health challenge that many nations around the world are currently grappling to tackle. A casual examination of the major public health campaigns globally is likely to reveal that many of them, particularly in developed countries, have placed the issue of childhood obesity prevention and intervention squarely on their agenda. Fueled by statistical reports and research asserting that the prevalence of overweight and obese children is on the rise, concern has steadily grown among authorities over the so-called childhood obesity epidemic.[1] According to recent data from the World Health Organization, there were more than 40 million overweight children under the age of five in 2011. In addition, this phenomenon is reportedly no longer confined to only high-income countries, with the World Health Organization further reporting that more than 30 million of these children are presently living in developing countries and 10 million in developed countries.[2] A similar trend has been observed in Australia, with one in four young people aged 5 to 17 reported to be overweight or obese in 2007–8, up four percentage points from 1995 (21%).[3] The recent statistic has also generally remained stable, as evident from the latest findings that estimate the prevalence of overweight and obese young Australians to be 25.3 percent.[4]

However, the best way of managing this apparent childhood obesity hysteria has divided parties such as policy makers, health professionals, educators, child activists, concerned members of the public, and the like. One camp has largely sought to stamp out what they perceive to be an increasingly worrisome societal problem by promoting and sanctioning the introduction of a myriad of prevention and intervention initiatives. Driven by beliefs that excess weight is a causative factor for a host of health problems, they have sought to intervene by placing an increasing amount of pressure on children who fall in the overweight or obese body mass index (BMI) percentile range to lose weight, such as by reducing their caloric intake and/or increasing their activity levels. One avenue through which they have attempted to exert their influence can be seen in antifat interventions in schools. On the other hand, other groups are concerned about the impact of this crusade to fight childhood obesity, arguing not only that the rationale behind it is flawed, but that these interventions are also hurting our children. With this in mind, the aims of this chapter are to discuss (1) case examples of antifat curriculum and initiatives in schools; (2) the arguments for such interventions; (3) the adverse effects of these school-based initiatives on children's physical and psychological well-being; (4) antifat interventions at a societal level; and (5) potential solutions and suggestions for future interventions.

CASE EXAMPLES OF ANTIFAT CURRICULUM AND INITIATIVES IN SCHOOLS

Australia-Based Strategies

In Australia, governments have embarked on a number of different initiatives at federal, state, and territory levels to address the issues of both adult and childhood obesity. For example, the National Preventative Health Taskforce was established in April 2008 to develop a National Preventative Health Strategy, which sought to outline proposals for interventions aimed at reducing the impact of three key areas of concern—obesity being one of them. Specifically, the strategy aims to "halt and reverse the rise in overweight and obesity in Australia by 2020" by setting the medium- to long-term goals of increasing the percentage of children and adults with "healthy body weight by 3% within 10 years," increasing the proportion of children and adults "meeting national guidelines for healthy eating and physical activity by 15% within 6 years," and helping to "assure Australian children a healthy start to life."[5] It also highlights a number of recommendations relating to school policies, such as that pertaining to the curriculum and nutrition guidelines, catering (including vending machines), the food and drink brought by children into school, physical activity, building layout and recreational facilities, and support and professional development for educators around implementing strategies.

The National Healthy School Canteens Project was commenced in 2008 to improve the quality of foods sold in Australian school canteens by developing national guidelines and training for canteen managers. Funded by the Australian government as part of the Australian Better Health Initiative, the project is based on nutritional guidelines such as *The Australian Guide to Healthy Eating and Dietary Guidelines for Children and Adolescents in Australia* and is driven by the underlying belief that the provision of accessible healthy and nutritious food would assist in combating the trend of childhood obesity.[6] Specifically, the strategy classifies food into three categories according to their nutritional value, similar to a traffic-light system: (1) green ("always on the canteen menu"—to be promoted highly and made available every day in the canteen), (2) amber ("select carefully"—to be promoted less and sold in smaller serving sizes), and (3) red ("not recommended on the canteen menu"—provided in strictly limited quantities). Across states, schools have since developed and implemented the project, including the Fresh Tastes Healthy School Canteen Strategy in New South Wales, the Smart Choices Healthy Food and Drink Supply Strategy for Queensland Schools, the Victorian Healthy Eating Enterprise in Victoria, and the Healthy Food and Drink Supply in Western Australia. As an extension to the strategy, the New South Wales government also implemented a ban on the sale of sugar-sweetened drinks in canteens and vending machines in government schools in 2007.[7]

Another program that has been introduced to target the incidence of childhood obesity is the Stephanie Alexander Kitchen Garden Program, which was introduced in 2001 and is currently being implemented in 297 primary schools across Australia. The combined cooking and gardening program, which provides children with the opportunity to grow, prepare, and eat fresh seasonal produce, aims to introduce pleasurable and memorable food education and experiences to children. It is also hoped that positively influencing children's food preferences and attitudes toward environmental sustainability would facilitate the cultivation of healthy, nutritious long-term eating habits in them.

School-Based Weight Screening and BMI Report Cards

The practice of sending children home to parents with a grade on their weight has clearly become a rising trend, as governments seek to flag children who they believe are at risk for weight-related health problems. In the United States for example, at least 19 states have since jumped on the BMI report card bandwagon, including California, Illinois, and Massachusetts (although not every state requires parents to be notified of the results).[8] Malaysia and the UK have also introduced a similar policy in their attempt to curb childhood obesity rates.[9] Largely driven by the belief that parents would be prompted to take the relevant measures to nip any potential or existing weight problems in their children if they were alerted to their children's weight status and its associated consequences, these BMI screening programs typically include an explanation of the findings from the weigh-in, recommendations for follow-up actions (if relevant), and suggestions on healthy eating habits, physical activity, and weight management.[10]

Singapore's Trim and Fit (TAF) Program

Perhaps one of the more infamous antifat school initiatives is the TAF program, which was implemented across primary- to pretertiary-level schools in Singapore from 1992 to 2007. Known for its heavy-handed approach to fighting childhood obesity (as well as the ironic fact that the acronym TAF spelled "fat" backwards, which consequently resulted in many a TAF program member becoming the source of fat jokes), the program subjected students who were classified overweight or obese (based on regular BMI measurement assessments) to additional activities designed to promote weight loss. These included a strict diet regiment, vigorous exercise or physical activities (on top of their regular physical education curriculum) that were organized during the recess break or outside school hours, and consultations with the school health service or the government's Health Promotion Board for more intensive follow-ups with doctors and dietitians.[11] There was also some variation among schools in how they chose to implement the other aspects of the program. In some schools, members of the TAF program were segregated by being made to sit at specified tables during recess to enable their food intake to be monitored; while in others, they had to wear "I'm Trim and Fit" wristbands. In addition, some schools issued this group of children "calorie cash," akin to food ration coupons representing caloric values that they were not allowed to exceed when purchasing food items. The amount of "calorie cash" received was also inversely proportional to the child's weight.[12] However, following increasing flak over the stigmatizing aspect of the program, it was eventually scrapped in 2007 and replaced with a holistic program aimed at improving fitness levels and psychological health that included students of all sizes.

Lunchbox Policies

In an attempt to further police children's diet and food choices, some schools have issued lunchbox policies to dictate what types of food children are encouraged or not allowed to bring to school. In Australia, for example, staff at kindergarten and child care centers double up as "nutritional watchdogs" to educate families on restricting "unhealthy" food and to check lunchboxes for any objectionable food items (which, when found, are promptly sent back home). Treats, such as birthday cakes and dessert, are also replaced with the more acceptable (and less calorie-filled) birthday badges, hat, and fruit.[13] A similar situation has also unfolded in the UK.[14]

ARGUMENTS FOR ANTIFAT CURRICULUM
AND INITIATIVES IN SCHOOLS

Proponents of antifat interventions in schools often cite their concerns about the short-term and long-term impact of obesity on children's well-being as a basis for putting forth their policies. In particular, they allude to the physical, psychological, and social problems linked with childhood obesity, such as type 2 diabetes, asthma, impaired immune function, high blood pressure, orthopedic complications, sleep disturbances, depression, poor self-esteem, and social discrimination. It has also been suggested that obese children are at a greater propensity for poorer health outcomes in adult life, including obesity, cardiovascular disease, insulin resistance, and heightened risk of mortality and morbidity.[15]

In addition, those who believe in the need to eradicate childhood obesity have pointed to research that has demonstrated positive outcomes in antifat school interventions as justification for continuing to push for more of such initiatives.[16] For example, it was recently reported that the rates of childhood obesity had declined in U.S. cities such as New York, Philadelphia, and Los Angeles from 2007 to 2011—a reverse in the trend that had been observed for decades. Although no specific reason for the decline could be established, authorities believed that the changes to the school curriculum as part of their efforts to target childhood obesity had played a role.[17] Further evidence that has been cited comes from an examination of antiobesity initiatives, including the introduction of BMI report cards, in the U.S. state of Arkansas. Specifically, findings from the three-year follow-up study indicated that BMI levels among the children and adolescents surveyed had reached a plateau. The study also argued that concerns over issues such as unhealthy weight control practices were generally unfounded, citing the absence of any increase in dieting behaviors, diet pill use, excessive exercise, or weight-related teasing.[18] Other researchers have even gone as far as to suggest that BMI screening and antifat interventions can be valuable and have its greatest impact in children as young as two years old, possibly because children at this developmental stage are more susceptible to change. Such recommendations have also cited behavioral weight management strategies such as limiting the consumption of juice drinks, switching to skim or low-fat nonflavored milk, and keeping a tally on the proportion of calories from added sugar and fat.[19]

ADVERSE IMPACT OF ANTIFAT CURRICULUM
AND INITIATIVES

Despite the apparent evidence and support for antifat curriculum and initiatives in schools, concerns have arisen over the risk that these interventions are inadvertently damaging children's psychological well-being due to their myopic focus on weight as an indicator of health and their zealous mission to eliminate the so-called problem around fatness. In particular, a number of studies have proposed that measures such as BMI screening and report cards, food policing, and differential treatment of fat schoolchildren have contributed to increased rates of disordered eating and body image dissatisfaction. For example, a recent study by the C.S. Mott Children's Hospital National Poll on Children's Health examined the relationship between school-based childhood obesity prevention programs (including nutrition education, restrictions on sweets or "junk food" in the classroom, BMI measurements, and incentives for exercise) and a rise in eating disorder symptomatology among children aged 6 to 14. The poll results demonstrated that 30 percent of parents reported at least one concerning behavior in their children that was possibly indicative of the development of an eating disorder, such as "inappropriate dieting, excessive worry about fat in foods, being preoccupied with food content or labels, refusing family meals, and having too much physical activity." In addition, 7 percent of parents provided feedback that their children had been made to feel guilty about the kind and amount of food they were consuming at school.[20] Another study in Canada similarly argued that such programs were having the unintended effect of triggering disordered eating and "creating sudden neuroses around food in children who never before worried about their weight." As Sharon Kirkey noted in a *National Post* article dated March 31, 2013, detailing the Canadian study, children undergoing puberty may be more likely to be vulnerable, given that the physical changes to their body (which often involve increased body fat) may be perceived as running contrary to the thin ideal celebrated in many societies. Children who display perfectionistic tendencies and constantly feel driven to strive for excellence may also be at higher risk for developing disordered eating, if they take the message about healthy lifestyles "to the extreme."[21]

These findings suggesting that antifat school interventions could potentially be a contributing factor for the development of disordered eating, body image disturbances, and poor self-worth would probably be regarded as unsurprising by some. In fact, research has demonstrated that fat children are usually already cognizant of their weight status and that they do desire to manage it, with a proportion of this group resorting to extreme weight control or loss measures to achieve their weight goals.[22] Given especially that many cultures tend to place thinness on a pedestal, children and adolescents may feel pressured to resort to such unhealthy weight management behaviors to conform to the "ideal." As such, antifat programs that draw further attention to fat children by embarrassingly singling them out and insinuating that they are a problem that requires fixing may very likely result in detrimental repercussions to their emotional and psychological well-being. Findings from retrospective studies conducted on the TAF program in Singapore clearly attest to the problematic nature of the weight-biased focus in these interventions. Lee and colleagues found in their research in 2005 that approximately 26.9 percent of the sample of 126 participants with anorexia nervosa, many of whom had been members of the TAF program, had cited weight-biased teasing and comments as precipitating factors for their eating disorder.[23] Another unpublished study of 4,400 female Singaporean students found that about 7 percent of them were at risk of developing eating disorders, and that out of this group, one-third had participated in the TAF program. In addition, 60 percent of the sample reported having been teased about their weight.[24] It is evident that there is a substantial body of research indicating that individual weight and body shape concerns, as well as the experience of being subjected to weight-related teasing factor highly in the development of eating disorder symptomatology and negative body image.[25] It is thus perplexing as to why antifat interventions that appear to be the breeding ground for such problems continue to be promoted, given that weight-biased initiatives may actually undermine health promotion efforts.[26] Moreover, fat children are not the only ones impacted by these interventions, with nonoverweight children and adolescents also having been found to have engaged in unhealthy weight control and/or weight loss practices.[27] Even a perception of being overweight among nonoverweight adolescents may contribute to greater weight gain.[28]

In addition, strategies that involve segregating and singling out fat children for intervention are more than likely to invite the problems of fat shaming and stigmatization. Children learn from an early age that culture generally frowns on fatness, so slapping the label of "overweight" or "obese" on them only serves to fuel the stigma associated with being fat.[29] Given that most children and adolescents are at the stage where fitting in and having a sense of belonging with their peer group becomes paramount, being socially rejected and isolated can lead to issues such as impaired self-esteem, self-blame, and depression.[30] Furthermore, shaming children into thinking that their bodies are somehow not "right" and need to be changed fails to take into consideration the diversity of shapes and sizes that bodies come in. Shaming is far from being an effective motivator for change—instead, it evokes fear, self-criticism, and self-loathing.[31] Studies have even found that drawing attention to their fatness can contribute to children feeling more sensitive and conscious about their bodies, which in turn can reduce the likelihood of them (particularly girls) participating in physical activities and sport.[32] Indeed, if shaming was such a valuable tactic, there would be no fat people around.

Paradoxically, there is a plethora of research suggesting that dieting predicts future weight gain, regardless of whether these individuals maintain their diet and/or exercise program.[33] To illustrate, a study that reviewed research on the long-term outcomes of calorie-restricting diets found although diets do result in short-term weight loss, dieters who manage to maintain their weight loss appear to be the "rare exception rather than the rule." In fact, one-third to two-thirds of dieters eventually regain more weight than they had lost on their diets. In addition, dieting was not associated with significant health benefits—and even when improvements were demonstrated, these could not be causally attributed to the effects of dieting. The authors further argued that methodological flaws in many of these studies very possibly resulted in an overestimation of the effectiveness of dieting in sustaining weight loss.[34] Similarly, research by the National Institutes of Health indicated that "one third to two thirds of the weight is regained within one year (after weight loss), and almost all is regained within five years."[35] It is also important to note that these findings are not limited to adult populations, with dietary restraint and extreme weight control measures having been found to predict obesity in adolescents.[36] One of the largest studies to demonstrate this phenomenon in adolescents is the Growing Up Today Study, a prospective study that surveyed a sample of more than 16,000 adolescents aged 9 to 14 years over a three-year period. Findings from the study indicated that both male and female adolescents who were "frequent dieters" (dieting two to seven days a week) and "infrequent dieters" (dieting less than once a month to once a week) had gained significantly more weight than nondieters at the end of the three years. The authors also concluded that the weight gain was likely to be attributed to the dieting behaviors, as they had factored out possible confounding factors such as age, BMI, physical development, physical activity, calorie intake, and height change.[37] Another study, Project Eating and Activity in Teens and Young Adults, similarly demonstrated that the strongest predictors of weight gain over a 10-year period in the sample population were dieting and unhealthy weight control behaviors, particularly missing meals, restrictive eating, and using food substitutes and diet pills.[38] As such, it is evident that the calorie control strategies recommended by many antifat school interventions not only may be futile in reversing obesity but may ironically also be contributing to it.

Another problematic aspect of antifat school-based interventions pertains to the fact that most have based the rationale for their strategies on the flawed premise that excess weight is inevitably a problem that needs to be solved by getting people to reduce their weight down to the "healthy" BMI range. Firstly, a growing body of research has demonstrated that fat is not necessarily synonymous with unhealthy and/or bad, in the same way that thin is not necessarily healthy and/or good.[39] While it is acknowledged that there is some association between increased body fat and a greater risk for physical health illnesses, and that an individual's health is more likely to be negatively affected if he or she is at the statistical extremes of either thinness or fatness, correlation does not necessarily imply causation. Contrary to the information we have been fed by health professionals who operate from the conventional weight-centered paradigm, studies have found that this risk for poorer health outcomes disappears or is significantly decreased after factors such as fitness and activity levels, dietary intake, socioeconomic status, and weight cycling are taken into account.[40] What is equally pertinent is the finding that engaging in healthy lifestyle behaviors is linked to reduced mortality risk levels, regardless of weight status.[41] Secondly, given the emphasis on BMI as a means of assessing health and wellness in these school-based programs, the BMI fallacy is one that certainly deserves mentioning. The BMI, which is calculated by dividing weight by height squared, was initially designed by Belgian mathematician, astronomer, and statistician Lambert Adolphe Jacques Quetelet as a statistical formula to measure the average body size of large populations. Ironically, it was never intended for use on a single individual. Moreover, the BMI is an inaccurate predictor of body fatness on an individual level, which in turn makes conclusions about a person's health, body composition, blood pressure, fitness level, mortality, and morbidity based on this highly dubious calculation.[42] Simply consider that Hollywood actors George Clooney and Tom Cruise fall in the "overweight" and "obese" category respectively, and you get the idea of how laughable the BMI tool probably is.[43] To add to the quandary, using the BMI measure with children is fraught with even more problems simply due to the fact that they would be experiencing weight fluctuations as part of their physical developmental process. As such, penalizing children for failing to land themselves in the "acceptable" weight category when their weight changes could quite possibly be part of a normal growth spurt benefits no one. An increasing number of concerned professionals have also argued that introducing BMI report cards does more harm than good, citing the dearth of research demonstrating that weight screening and report cards are effective in reducing the rates of childhood obesity.[44] Other potential problems highlighted include the question over whether parents and children understand and appreciate the consequences of the reported results enough to take the recommended action, possible feelings of self-blame among parents over their children's weight, and the role of cultural, ethnic, and socioeconomic status differences in influencing weight.[45]

Despite some research findings arguing for the effectiveness and success of antifat school initiatives, other studies have failed to demonstrate similar results. In particular, the evidence suggests that these interventions have not been significantly effective in preventing or reversing weight gain.[46] A research publication issued by the Australian government, for example, reported that "there is also very little high-quality evidence on the effectiveness of obesity prevention programs for young children. Studies on the impact of diet and physical activity programs have produced inconsistent results, and Australian research has found that managing obesity through general practice is expensive and there is little evidence that it is effective."[47] Nonetheless, it is also worthwhile to note that a number of these interventions have had some success in improving lifestyle behaviors, such as those related to nutrition and increased physical activity.[48] As such, given the generally limited support for a weight-based approach to managing childhood obesity, it would be beneficial to shift to a health-based paradigm that incorporates a holistic view of well-being.

Finally, by being fixated on eliminating obesity and focusing interventions only on fat children, schools run the risk of ignoring the nutrition, physical activity, and health needs of thinner and nonoverweight students. Potential issues of concern such as malnutrition, eating disorders, fatigue, impaired immune system, and menstruation problems may also be missed.

ANTIFAT INTERVENTIONS AT A SOCIETAL LEVEL

Interventions targeting fat children are not confined to the realm of schools, as evident from the recent proliferation of community campaigns and initiatives designed around weight-based goals. Unfortunately, many of these have also incorporated elements of antifat messages in them. Perhaps a clear example of this can be seen in the most recent season of the reality show *The Biggest Loser*, where fat young people were teamed up with their fat parents to compete with other teams in losing the most amount of weight for prize money. However, the show, which prides itself on promoting health, appears to be a public spectacle of socially sanctioned shaming where bodies that are considered to have failed to fit in with the acceptable "norm" are paraded on television to be vilified nationally under the guise of improving health and promoting weight loss.[49] Other antiobesity campaigns in the United States that have ignited controversy include the Strong4Life campaign in Georgia and the Better Example campaign in Minnesota, which incorporated images of fat children, as well as the recent advertisement in California that digitally altered an image of a young girl to make her appear fatter.[50] Even the initiative of the wife of current U.S. president Barack Obama, Michelle Obama, to reduce the prevalence of childhood obesity in the United States came under fire after her campaign was regarded as marginalizing fat children and "turning them into targets."[51] One could be forgiven for wondering what messages we are potentially sending to our children if we continue to myopically focus on efforts on getting that number on the scale down to a socially acceptable range.

SOLUTIONS AND RECOMMENDATIONS FOR FUTURE INTERVENTIONS

In light of the potentially adverse impact of antifat curriculum and initiatives on children's physical, psychological, and social well-being, as well as the limited support for its effectiveness in managing childhood obesity, it is evident that these interventions (although generally well intentioned) are causing harm. A weight-based approach appears to have limited merit in efforts to control or reduce weight, particularly in the long term, as evident from the dismal success rates of dieting and the propensity for dieters to regain the weight lost (and more). Even more worryingly, these so-called healthy living school-based programs have been associated with disordered eating, unhealthy weight management behaviors, body image dissatisfaction, poor self-worth, depression, and weight-based teasing and shaming. It is thus imperative that we shift our focus away from the conventionally narrow-minded approach where assumptions about our health are made based solely on the number on the scale, to a more holistic health-based paradigm that accepts and includes a diversity of body shapes and sizes. To illustrate, the following are examples of recommendations for future school-based interventions that could prove beneficial:

- Adopt a weight-neutral, health-based approach that refrains from targeting only fat children and focusing on weight modification goals. This would involve structuring school programs such as physical activities around promoting health for all children and adolescents regardless of shape and size. In particular, interventions should focus on behaviors that are amenable to modification, such as self-care skills, physical activity, time spent watching television, and bullying. Correspondingly, weight is not a behavior and is therefore not an appropriate target for change.[52]

- Avoid using language that has overt or covert antifat messages, such as "fat is bad," "eradicate," and "problem," which may inadvertently foster fat stigma and discrimination. Using "diet" language, such as "good foods" and "bad foods," is also unhelpful as it can set children up to think of foods in a moralistic way, which in turn could trigger conflict and feelings of guilt when eating. Instead, discuss food as "fuel for the body" and our bodies as vehicles that require the "fuel" to function effectively. Teaching children to be more aware of and honor their body's internal cues (that is, differentiating between physiological hunger and satiety signals, and external cues that may also trigger eating) can also be useful.[53]

- Focus on providing sufficient opportunities for encouraging appropriate levels of physical activity for health and pleasure, rather than weight control or loss.

- Acknowledge and accept that bodies come in a diversity of shapes and sizes, while celebrating individual uniqueness. As such, setting expectations and goals around getting children to fall in the so-called healthy

BMI range is only one part of the equation to improving health and fails to recognize that health encompasses many other aspects.

- Include strategies related to promoting positive body image in the curriculum. These may include developing media literacy by raising awareness of the generally limited representation of body shapes and sizes in the media and teaching children to be of critical of the messages they are exposed to; acknowledging diversity in people; celebrating individuality; and shifting the focus away from weight.
- Implement and enforce policies to target issues of weight-based teasing and bullying in schools. Teaching respect for body size diversity to children can also be beneficial.
- Recognize the role of parents in encouraging positive health behaviors at home and provide support to help them promote such behaviors at home where necessary.

CONCLUSION

Policy makers, health professionals, educators, and other relevant parties have the power to nurture our children's physical, psychological, and social development, as well as enhance their overall well-being. The school provides ample opportunity for this to occur and great care should be taken to ensure that any interventions introduced are in the best interest of our children and adolescents. In light of the potential harm antifat curriculum and initiatives could result in, a new way of thinking about health is needed—in particular, one that moves away from the conventional weight-based approach to a holistic perspective that encompasses all other aspects of health.

NOTES

1. Based on the BMI-for-age growth charts for children and adolescents aged 2 to 20 years old developed by the Centers for Disease Control and Prevention in the United States, individuals in the 85th to less than 95th percentile range are categorized as "overweight" while those at the 95th percentile or greater are classified "obese."

2. "Overweight and Obesity," World Health Organization, last modified March 2013, http://www.who.int/mediacentre/factsheets/fs311/en/.

3. "Feature Article 1: Children Who Are Overweight or Obese," Australian Bureau of Statistics, June 4, 2010, http://www.abs.gov.au/AUSSTATS/abs@.nsf/Lookup/1301.0Chapter11062009-10.

4. "Australian Health Survey: First Results, 2011–12," Australian Bureau of Statistics, October 29, 2012, http://www.abs.gov.au/ausstats/abs@.nsf/Lookup/4364.0.55.001Chapter1002011-12.

5. "National Preventative Health Strategy: The Roadmap for Action," National Preventative Health Task Force, June 30, 2009, http://www.preventativehealth.org

.au/internet/preventativehealth/publishing.nsf/Content/CCD7323311E358BECA257 5FD000859E1/$File/nphs-roadmap.pdf.

6. "National Healthy School Canteens: Guidelines for Healthy Foods and Drinks Supplied in School Canteens," Australian Government Department of Health and Ageing, June 2010, http://www.health.gov.au/internet/main/publishing.nsf/content/ E957A2FD2F25C36BCA2574830007BAF2/$File/Guidelines%20for%20healthy %20foods%20and%20drinks%20supplied%20in%20school%20canteens.pdf.

7. "Sugar Sweetened Drink Ban for NSW Schools," NSW Government of Health, August 31, 2006, http://www0.health.nsw.gov.au/pubs/2006/softdrink_ban.html.

8. Julie Deardorff, "BMI Measuring in Schools Proves Weighty Issue," *Chicago Tribune*, May 17, 2013, http://articles.chicagotribune.com/2013-05-17/health/ct-met -bmi-backlash-20130517_1_bmi-childhood-obesity-rates-muscular-people.

9. Tamara Baluja and Kate Hammer, "Are Schools Going Too Far in Measuring Student BMI and Banning Junk Food?," *Globe and Mail*, last modified March 7, 2013, http://www.theglobeandmail.com/news/national/education/are-schools-going -too-far-in-measuring-student-bmi-and-banning-junk-food/article4209904/.

10. Allison J. Nihiser et al., "BMI Measurement in Schools," *Pediatrics* 124 (2009): 89–97, doi:10.1542/peds.2008-3586L.

11. Cheong Mui Toh, Jeffrey Cutter, and Suok Kai Chew, "School Based Intervention Has Reduced Obesity in Singapore," *British Medical Journal* 324, no. 7334 (2002): 427–30, doi:10.1136/bmj.324.7334.427/a.

12. "Obesity Series Part III: Singapore," PRI's *The World*, November 14, 2007, http://www.pri.org/theworld/?q=node/14022.

13. " 'Kindy Police' to Patrol Lunches," *Gold Coast News*, May 20, 2009, http:// www.goldcoast.com.au/article/2009/05/20/80521_gold-coast-news.html.

14. Julie Gunlock, "National Review: Food Police and Lunchbox Privacy," July 22, 2010, http://www.npr.org/templates/story/story.php?storyId=128687780.

15. C. M. Doak et al., "The Prevention of Overweight and Obesity in Children and Adolescents: A Review of Interventions and Programmes," *Obesity Reviews* 7 (2006): 111–36, doi:10.1111/j.1467-789X.2006.00234.x; Centre for Community Child Health, "Preventing Overweight and Obesity: Practice Resource," accessed June 18, 2013, http://www.rch.org.au/uploadedFiles/Main/Content/ccch/PR_Prevent_OO_all.pdf.

16. M. Story, "School-Based Approaches for Preventing and Treating Obesity," *International Journal of Obesity* 23, suppl. 2 (1999): 43–51, http://gsareach.com/ wp-content/uploads/2009/11/Story-School-Obesity-3.pdf; Paul J. Veugelers and Angela L. Fitzgerald, "Effectiveness of School Programs in Preventing Childhood Obesity: A Multilevel Comparison," *American Journal of Public Health* 95, no. 3 (2005), doi:10.2105/AJPH.2004.045898.

17. Sabrina Tavernise, "Obesity in Young Is Seen as Falling in Several Cities," NYTimes.com, last modified December 13, 2012, http://www.nytimes.com/2012/12/ 11/health/childhood-obesity-drops-in-new-york-and-philadelphia.html?pagewante-d=all&_r=2&; Sydney Lupkin, "Philadelphia Students Slimmer; Schools' Anti-Obesity Efforts Cited," ABC News, September 11, 2012, http://abcnews.go.com/ Health/philadelphia-school-children-slim-data-shows-obesity-reduced/story? id=17210143#.Uc03JBxKDF9.

18. J. M. Raczynski et al., "Arkansas Act 1220 of 2003 to Reduce Childhood Obesity: Its Implementation and Impact on Child and Adolescent Body Mass Index," *Journal of Public Health Policy* 30, suppl. 1 (2009): 124–40, doi:10.1057/jphp.2008.54.

19. Katherine Hobson, "Study: Anti-Obesity Program Works Best in Youngest Kids," *Wall Street Journal Health Blog*, May 6, 2011, http://blogs.wsj.com/health/2011/05/06/study-anti-obesity-program-works-best-in-youngest-kids/; Joseph Brownstein, "Childhood Obesity Best Battled in Schools, Research Finds," Live Science, December 6, 2011, http://www.livescience.com/36017-childhood-obesity-interventions-schools.html.

20. University of Michigan Health System, "School Obesity Programs May Promote Worrisome Eating Behaviors and Physical Activity in Kids," *ScienceDaily*, January 27, 2012, http://www.sciencedaily.com/releases/2012/01/120124151207.htm.

21. Sharon Kirkey, "School-Based 'Healthy Living' Programs Triggering Eating Disorders in Some Children: Canadian Study," *National Post*, March 31, 2013, http://life.nationalpost.com/2013/03/31/school-based-healthy-living-programs-triggering-eating-disorders-in-some-children-canadian-study/.

22. Dianne Neumark-Sztainer et al., "Weight-Related Concerns and Behaviors among Overweight and Nonoverweight Adolescents," *Archives of Pediatric and Adolescent Medicine* 156, no. 2 (2002): 171–78, doi:10.1001/archpedi.156.2.171.

23. H. Y. Lee et al., "Anorexia Nervosa in Singapore: An Eight-Year Retrospective Study," *Singapore Medical Journal* 46, no. 6 (2005): 275–81, http://www.ncbi.nlm.nih.gov/pubmed/15902355.

24. Sandra Davie, "School Link to Eating Disorders Possible," *Straits Times*, May 16, 2005, http://www.moe.gov.sg/media/forum/2005/forum_letters/20050520.pdf.

25. Joel D. Killen et al., "Pursuit of Thinness and Onset of Eating Disorder Symptoms in a Community Sample of Adolescent Girls: A Three-Year Prospective Analysis," *International Journal of Eating Disorders* 16, no. 3 (1994): 227–38, doi:10.1002/1098-108X(199411)16:3<227:AID-EAT2260160303>3.0.CO;2-L; M. Sharma, "School-Based Interventions for Childhood and Adolescent Obesity," *Obesity Reviews* 7, no. 3 (2006): 261–69, doi:10.1111/j.1467-789X.2006.00227.x.

26. Maho Isono, Patti Lou Watkins, and Lee Ee Lian, "Bon Bon Fatty Girl: A Qualitative Exploration of Weight Bias in Singapore," in *The Fat Studies Reader*, ed. Esther Rothblum and Sondra Solovay (New York: New York University Press, 2009), 127–38.

27. Jillian Croll et al., "Prevalence and Risk and Protective Factors Related to Disordered Eating Behaviors among Adolescents: Relationship to Gender and Ethnicity," *Journal of Adolescent Health* 31, no. 2 (2002): 166–75, doi:10.1016/S1054-139X(02)00368-3.

28. Koenraad Cuypers et al., "Being Normal Weight but Feeling Overweight in Adolescence May Affect Weight Development into Young Adulthood —an 11-Year Followup: The HUNT Study, Norway," *Journal of Obesity* (2012), doi:10.1155/2012/601872.

29. M. B. Schwartz and R. Puhl, "Childhood Obesity: A Societal Problem to Solve," *Obesity Reviews* 4 (2003): 57–71, doi:10.1046/j.1467-789X.2003.00093.x.

30. Joanne P. Ikeda, Patricia B. Crawford, and Gail Woodward-Lopez, "BMI Screening in Schools: Helpful or Harmful?," *Health Education Research* 21, no. 6 (2006): 761–69, doi: 10.1093/her/cyl144.

31. "Stigmatizing Obese Individuals Is the Wrong Way to Address Obesity," Yale Rudd Center for Food Policy and Obesity, January 24, 2013, http://www.yale ruddcenter.org/stigmatizing-obese-individuals-is-the-wrong-way-to-address-obesity; Rebecca M. Puhl and Chelsea A. Heuer, "Obesity Stigma: Important Considerations for Public Health," *American Journal of Public Health* 100, no. 6 (2010): 1019–28, doi:10.2105/AJPH.2009.159491.

32. Jennifer A. O'Dea, "Prevention of Child Obesity: 'First, Do No Harm,' " *Health Education Research* 20, no. 2 (2005): 259–65, doi:10.1093/her/cyg116.

33. Linda Bacon and Lucy Aphramor, "Weight Science: Evaluating the Evidence for a Paradigm Shift," *Nutrition Journal* 10, no. 9 (2011), doi:10.1186/1475-2891-10 -9; W. C. Miller, "How Effective Are Traditional Dietary and Exercise Interventions for Weight Loss?," *Medicine and Science in Sports and Exercise* 31, no. 8 (1999): 1129–34, doi:10.1097/00005768-199908000-00008.

34. Traci Mann et al., "Medicare's Search for Effective Obesity Treatments," *American Psychologist* 62, no. 3 (2007): 220–33, doi:10.1037/0003-066X.62.3.220.

35. National Institutes of Health, "Methods for Voluntary Weight Loss and Control (Technology Assessment Conference Panel)," *Annals of Internal Medicine* 116 (1992): 942–49.

36. Eric Stice et al., "Psychological and Behavioral Risk Factors for Obesity Onset in Adolescent Girls: A Prospective Study," *Journal of Consulting and Clinical Psychology* 73, no. 2 (2005): 195–202, doi:10.1037/0022-006X.73.2.195; Alison E. Field et al., "Relation between Dieting and Weight Change among Preadolescents and Adolescents," *Pediatrics* 112, no. 4 (2003): 900–906, doi:10.1542/peds.112.4.900; "Adolescent Dieting May Predict Obesity and Eating Disorders," American Dietetic Association, last modified October 11, 2012, http://www.rxpgnews.com/obesity/ Adolescent_Dieting_May_Predict_Obesity_and_Eating__3907_3907.shtml.

37. Field et al., "Relation between Dieting and Weight Change."

38. Dianne Neumark-Sztainer et al., "Dieting and Unhealthy Weight Control Behaviors during Adolescence: Associations with 10-Year Changes in Body Mass Index," *Journal of Adolescent Health* 50, no. 1 (2012): 80–86, doi:10.1016/ j.jadohealth.2011.05.010.

39. Alexandra Sifferlin, "Can You Be Fat and Fit—or Thin and Unhealthy?," *Time*, September 5, 2012, http://healthland.time.com/2012/09/05/can-you-be-fat-and-fit-or- thin-and-unhealthy/; Ernest Dempsey, "Op-Ed: No Evidence Weight Loss Improves Health, Says Nutrition Expert," *Digital Journal*, March 16, 2013, http://www .digitaljournal.com/article/345802; Alice Park, "Why Being Thin Doesn't Always Mean Being Healthy," *Time*, June 27, 2011, http://healthland.time.com/2011/06/27/ why-being-thin-doesnt-always-mean-being-healthy/.

40. Bacon and Aphramor, "Weight Science."

41. Eric M. Matheson, Dana E. King, and Charles J. Everett, "Healthy Lifestyle Habits and Mortality in Overweight and Obese Individuals," *Journal of the American Board of Family Medicine* 25, no. 1 (2012): 9–15, doi:10.3122/jabfm.2012.01.110164.

42. Jon Robison, "The HAES Files: Is the Body Mass Index a Good Measure of Health?," *Health at Every Size Blog*, October 24, 2011, http://healthateverysizeblog .org/2011/10/24/the-haes-files-is-the-body-mass-index-a-good-measure-of-health/.

43. Keith Devlin, "Do You Believe in Fairies, Unicorns, or the BMI?," Association for Size Diversity and Health, accessed June 25, 2013, https://sizediversityandhealth .org/content.asp?id=34&articleID=177.

44. Allison J. Nihiser et al., "BMI Measurement in Schools," *Pediatrics* 124 (2009): 89–97, doi:10.1542/peds.2008-3586L; Lauren Vogel, "The Skinny on BMI Report Cards," *Canadian Medical Association Journal* 183, no. 12 (2011): 787–88, doi:10.1503/cmaj.109-3927; E. W. Evans and K. R. Sonneville, "BMI Report Cards: Will They Pass or Fail in the Fight against Pediatric Obesity?," *Current Opinion Pediatrics* 21, no. 4 (2009): 231–36, doi:10.1097/MOP.0b013e32832ce04c.

45. C. Meghan McMurty and Elissa Jelalian, "Reporting Body Mass Index in the Schools: Are We Missing the Mark?," *Brown University Child and Adolescent Behavior Letter* 26, no. 1 (2010), http://www.bradleyhasbroresearch.org/oth/Page.asp?Page ID=OTH131026.

46. "Western Australian Obesity Think-Tank Background Paper," February 28, 2007, http://cbrcc.curtin.edu.au/reports_technical_reports/070219.pdf; Jasmine Antoine, "Where to from Here for Australian Childhood Obesity?," *Australian Medical Student Journal* 3, no.2 (2012): 20–23, http://www.amsj.org/archives/2447; Janet James, Peter Thomas, and David Kerr, "Preventing Childhood Obesity: Two-Year Follow-Up Results from the Christchurch Obesity Prevention Programme in Schools (CHOPPS)," *British Medical Journal* 335 (2007): 762–65, doi: http://dx.doi .org/10.1136/bmj.39342.571806.55.

47. Anne-marie Boxall, "Obesity Prevention in Young Children: What Does the Evidence Say?," Parliament of Australia Research Publications, May 1, 2009, http:// www.aph.gov.au/About_Parliament/Parliamentary_Departments/Parliamentary _Library/pubs/BN/0809/ObesityChildren#_Toc228928638.

48. Australian Government Productivity Commission, "Effectiveness of Obesity-Related Interventions," in *Childhood Obesity: An Economic Perspective*, October 25, 2010, http://www.pc.gov.au/__data/assets/pdf_file/0013/103315/07-chapter5.pdf.

49. Yoni Freedhoff, "So Long as the Biggest Loser Exploits Children, I'll Be Boycotting Its Advertisers' Products," Weighty Matters, January 2, 2013, http://www .weightymatters.ca/2013/01/so-long-as-biggest-loser-exploits.html.

50. Kathy Lohr, "Controversy Swirls around Harsh Anti-Obesity Ads," *NPR*, January 9, 2012, http://www.npr.org/2012/01/09/144799538/controversy-swirls-around-harsh-anti-obesity-ads; Lindsay Abrams, "Think of the (Fat) Children: Minnesota's 'Better Example' Anti-Obesity Campaign," *The Atlantic*, September 24, 2012, http://www.theatlantic.com/health/archive/2012/09/think-of-the-fat-children-minnesotas-better-example-anti-obesity-campaign/262674/; The Fat Chick Sings, "California Gov. Health Organization 'Photoshops' Kids Picture to Fight Childhood Obesity," June 5, 2013, http://fatchicksings.com/2013/06/05/california -gov-health-organization-photoshops-kids-picture-to-fight-childhood-obesity/.

51. Andrew Herzog, "First Lady's Anti-Obesity Campaign Turned Heavy Children into Targets, Group Says," cnsnews.com, August 11, 2011, http://www.cnsnews.com/

news/article/first-ladys-anti-obesity-campaign-turned-heavy-children-targets-group
-says.

52. Sigrun Danielsdottir, Deb Burgard, and Wendy Oliver-Pyatt, "AED Guidelines for Childhood Obesity Prevention Programs," Academy for Eating Disorders, accessed June 29, 2013, http://www.aedweb.org/AM/Template.cfm?Section=Advocacy &Template=/CM/ContentDisplay.cfm&ContentID=1659.

53. Body Positive, "Children and Weight: The Dilemmas," last modified March 5, 2011, http://www.bodypositive.com/childwt.htm.

14

The Fat Academy: Does Being Big Keep You from Getting Big in Scholarship?

Brittany Lockard

To most people reading this chapter, even to fat or size activists, this question probably seems fairly minor, or even irrelevant. After all, academia is an elite province, with only about 1.5 million professors (both full- and part-time) in the United States—or about 0.005 percent of the country's population.[1] My own field, art history, is still more rarified, with approximately 4,000 art or architectural historians in all of the United States, or roughly 0.003 percent of that 0.005 percent.[2] Academics make up a tiny fraction of 1 percent of the entire country; however, our impact on that larger population can be enormous. College professors frame the narratives their students hear and the discussions in which they engage. Scholars set the terms of our debates about everything from poetry to history to biology, and their discourse trickles down and becomes part of the way we conceptualize the world (just think about how frequently Freud's ideas still pop up in everyday contexts). Art historians curate our culture and decide which artists are relevant, whose images we will see, and who will be excluded from the museum and the canon. The more diverse the population of scholars, the more diverse the knowledge passed on, and the more inclusionary the scholarship.

IS THERE BIAS IN ACADEMIA?

The first question to ask, then, becomes "is there bias in academia?" I will admit that, even while working on my master's degree, I still thought academics were beyond ordinary bias. Academia invented intersectionality, I thought. We embrace gender studies, disability studies, identity studies, Chican@ studies, and so on. We spend years of our lives learning to question, to think critically and rationally. And then I experienced bias firsthand, and I also witnessed it happen to others. For instance, while eating dinner with a married couple and a fellow graduate student, the (admittedly inebriated) wife said that her department wouldn't need to hire people like my (nonwhite, Muslim) friend if they didn't "have" to teach the Qu'ran. She followed up on this statement by pointing out to my friend, "Once we stop teaching the Qu'ran, you're out of there!" To my shame, I said nothing at the time, paralyzed by shock and my deep awareness of the hierarchal differences between myself and the speaker.

Going beyond anecdata and looking at this issue more objectively is difficult, because parity between academic candidates (for jobs, fellowships, etc.) is hard to assess. Which school a candidate attended (for college, master's, and doctorate), what her field of study is (within art history, for example, you might specialize in areas as disparate as seventeenth-century French painting or contemporary Chinese sculpture) and her minor fields of study are, her mentors, her publication and conference presentation history, her employment, will all differentiate her from other candidates, making a one-to-one comparison problematic. Moreover, relatively few studies exist to determine the answer to this question, and those that do focus largely on (cis)gender to the exclusion of race, sexuality, age, body size, able-bodiedness, etc.

Straightforward statistics on the composition of American universities would suggest that my personal experiences of cultural bias in the ivory tower are closer to the rule than the exception. According to the U.S. Department of Education, in 2009 white faculty members comprised 79 percent of postsecondary educators, and 42 percent of educators were both white and male. Furthermore, the higher the status of the professor (tenure track rather than adjunct, associate rather than assistant, full tenure rather than associate) and the higher the pay, the whiter and more male the group became.[3] Moreover, the studies about academic bias that do exist further emphasize that scholars do not differ significantly from their counterparts in the general population in regards to bias. For instance, in 2012 Yale University performed an experiment on academic scientists (about 100), both male and female. They presented these researchers with one of two identical resumes, ostensibly from an undergraduate seeking a position as a lab manager. The only thing that changed on the resume was the gender of the name—one version sported a male name, the other a female. In the end, both men and women science faculty were more likely to hire the male student. They also ranked him higher in competency and were willing to pay him $4,000 more than the woman. Equally important for future career progression, they demonstrated more willingness to provide mentoring to the male than to the female candidate.[4] Thus even in a discipline composed of highly educated individuals deeply invested in critical thinking, subtle and inherent biases against women appear.

Gender discrimination in the academic world isn't limited to faculty in the sciences, however. Students exhibit gender discrimination; a 2000 study showed that when critical of their students, female university faculty members received harsher teaching evaluations than those of their male counterparts, irrespective of the gender of the students writing them.[5] Advisors also demonstrate gender bias against their advisees—a 2003 study found that letters of recommendation for female faculty applicants are shorter, contain fewer descriptions of their research accomplishments, give more emphasis to their teaching ability, and raise more doubts compared with letters written for their male counterparts.[6]

In one particularly relevant study, researchers took two actual curricula vitae (CV) from the same person (at different times in her career) and sent them to a random sample of university psychology departments, changing only the name (sometimes male and sometimes female) and asked faculty members to evaluate the applicant on a number of dimensions. The first CV was the version the actual applicant had used to get a job as a new assistant professor, and the second CV was the (more impressive) version she used years later as a candidate for tenure. The researchers found that when the first CV featured a male name, both male and female reviewers judged the candidate worthy of hire approximately 73 percent of the time. When the same CV used a female name, reviewers judged the candidate worthy of hire only 45 percent of the time. Furthermore, all participants more positively evaluated the research, teaching, and service contributions of the male job applicant over the female job applicant, even with an identical record.[7]

Review of the second (more impressive) tenure version of the vitae elicited no significant gender differences in ratings, although participants wrote four times as many cautionary or negative comments in the margins of their rating sheets for the female applicant, such as "We would have to see her job talk," or "I would need to see evidence that she had gotten these grants and publications on her own."[8] The fact that the reviewers rated the male and female tenure versions of the vitae more similarly than the new assistant professor versions suggests that women may be at greater risk of experiencing discrimination when information about their job qualifications is ambiguous. Of course, clear qualification does not eliminate all forms of bias against women: other research has shown that women who appear especially competent tend to be disliked at work and are penalized in other ways when they succeed.[9]

Although to the best of my knowledge, no studies explicitly demonstrate antifat bias in academia, a large body of work demonstrates antifat bias in American culture more generally. The lead researcher for a recent study published in the *International Journal of Obesity* investigating fat women's potential as employees noted that "strong obesity discrimination was displayed across all job selection criteria, such as starting salary, leadership potential, and likelihood of selecting an obese candidate for the job."[10] A study of actual earnings of fat individuals supports this conclusion, finding that fat workers suffer a wage penalty of 1.4 to 4.5 percent, with women suffering greater income disparity.[11] Two others suggest even greater wage loss.[12] Repeated studies have shown that physicians feel less empathetic toward their fat patients than their thin patients.[13] The general public responds strongly to cultural messages about fat: in a survey conducted by Yale University's Rudd Center for Food Policy and Obesity, almost half the participants indicated that they would rather lose a year off their lives than be fat. Between 15 and 30 percent of those participants would prefer to lose their marriages, become barren, be clinically depressed, or be alcoholic rather than be fat.[14] In fact, antifat bias is so pervasive that in 2008, members of the Mississippi Legislature actually introduced a bill to prohibit restaurants from serving food to fat people.[15] The ubiquity of antifat bias in the United States suggests that, as with gender bias, antifat bias also exists in academia.

CRITICAL SCHOLARS, CRITICAL SCHOLARSHIP

Fat scholars (as with fat people in general) face certain economic barriers that their thinner counterparts do not have to address, especially early in their careers.[16] Becoming a successful academic and scholar requires a fair amount of travel: to engage in original research, to present papers at conferences, to do campus interviews, etc. Graduate students and recent graduates, unless they have significant familial financial support, typically hover near the poverty line. Affording one airline ticket can strain or even break a budget; purchasing two airline tickets (as many people of size, myself included, must do) can be completely unfeasible.[17] Even if help is provided, the fat scholar can find herself in an awkward position. How do you compose a budget for a travel grant when you need two seats? How do you address this with the person scheduling your campus interview (and therefore paying for your ticket)? I also find it extremely difficult to find affordable and reasonably attractive "professional" clothing in plus sizes,[18] although my experience might not hold true for smaller fat people, such as "inbetweenies."[19]

Beyond an extra financial burden, fat scholars also face an insistent focus on their embodiment in their efforts toward contributing to scholarship in their fields. It has become almost customary for authors writing fat scholarship to discuss their own size, in the introduction, conclusion, or body of their text. Many seminal books include a first-person narrative about the author's own body. In *The Obesity Myth*, Paul Campos writes about his own weight and weight loss both in the final paragraph of his introduction and in the final chapter of his book.[20] Laura Fraser devotes the first several pages of the introduction of *Losing It* to her own struggles with fat and body image.[21] Richard Klein discusses not only his own but also his mother's and sister's preoccupation with fat in the preface to *Eat Fat*.[22] The introduction of Marilyn

Wann's *Fat!So?* is devoted to her own experiences as a fat woman,[23] and Shelley Bovey peppers *The Forbidden Body* with anecdotes from her own life.[24]

Many of these narratives possess a confessional tone, an "I should really mention . . ." air. Why should these authors feel the need to personally position themselves in relationship to fat? Perhaps they felt the need to do so for the same reason that on the very day that the art history department at the University of Kansas approved my dissertation proposal, giving me permission to pursue my fat-centered scholarly inquiries, a faculty member felt compelled to usher me into her office and give me some advice. She suggested that I change my topic away from the fat female nude in contemporary art. She cautioned that, as a fat woman writing about fat women, it would be difficult for me to give papers at panels or to find a job (once a hiring committee got a good look at me). She said that everyone would think I was too emotionally invested in my topic to write about it objectively. At the time, I was baffled by this exchange. Why should my appearance affect my research? Why should a member of a marginalized group be prevented from studying and writing about that marginalized group? In other words: what business of hers was my body?

In the years since this exchange occurred, I have seen the scenarios about which my professor cautioned me played out in real life. I once participated in a conference in which my panel had three speakers: myself, a fat white woman talking about photographs of fat, nude female bodies; a non-gender-conforming white person talking about transgender vlogs; and an (apparently) cisgender white man discussing "dime-store Indian" sculptures. At the end of the three presentations, the audience asked questions of us. Both myself and the non-gender-conforming participant had to answer questions about our identities, our physical bodies, and our relationship to our work. For instance, one woman asked whether or not I was a fat activist and if I felt like that impacted my scholarship (at a different conference, I was asked if *I* would be comfortable posing nude—upon receipt of this bizarre question, I felt rather as if I had actually been stripped nude right there; I was no longer an expert sharing my research, but merely a fat body on display).[25] However, the white male participant was asked only questions that directly related to his topic, as if his race/gender/etc. had no bearing or influence on the direction of his inquiry. He was allowed to speak with a disembodied, authoritative, neutral, and objective voice, while the non-gender-conforming participant and I were seen as contingent, embodied, emotionally invested. The cisgender white male is thus a default position; because I visibly differ from it, audiences continually interrogate my difference. I have had this same experience multiple times, and witnessed it happen to others again and again.

Sometimes the assumed primacy of the white male subject is hinted at subtly, as when I attended a conference panel about *feminist* art, in which all five participants were women—and yet the first question was asked by an older

white man, before the (female) moderator could even finish her call for questions. This man felt that, even in a space dominated by women and dedicated
to women's art, he had the right to speak first and loudest. Sometimes the
embodied nature of nonwhite men is made obvious, as when a woman attending a lecture at a small university felt comfortable asking personal questions
about the name and ethnicity of a scholar of Mexican art because the scholar's
surname was Japanese and she appeared to be Asian American. Since the
scholar presented neither as white nor as Latina in appearance, the audience
member thought she had no "obvious" reason to be interested in the subject
matter.

What this focus on the embodiment of marginalized academics does is
obfuscate the fact that cisgender white men are no more objective than anyone else. Standing on the outside, looking in on a marginalized group guaran-
tees only a different perspective, not objectivity;[26] both people are still on the
same street, in the same town (to unpardonably stretch my metaphor).
Everyone experiences disparate influences over the course of his life, and each
person is unique, but we all still exist in the same larger culture with the
subtle, intersecting, kyriarchal[27] pressures of misogyny, racism, and so on.

Do I have a complicated emotional relationship with fat and the body?
From the moment my parents placed my eight-year-old self on my first diet
to my embrace of fat activism in the current day. Have I experienced antifat
bias in my own life? Like many other fat people, I have been mocked, mooed
at, and insulted to my face, by friends, family, and complete strangers. My own
brother, who probably does not even recall this incident, called me "ham hock
thighs" for a brief period when I was in high school. And though some of my
experiences are unusual, I think that overall, the shame and pain in my past
are more common than they are unique. Being fat does not give me a special
window into Western attitudes about the body. It does not place me in a privileged location to speak about the body. Neither does being thin afford a special advantage to scholars. Antifat prejudice affects everyone in different
ways, and even women who adhere to idealized body norms can suffer on its
account and gain benefit from the work that fat activists and fat theorists are
doing.

I also suspect that my experience as a fat scholar working on fat theory is
not that different from fat scholars working on other, nonfat topics.
Although I don't have much firsthand knowledge about presenting research
that is nonfat related, I do have experience teaching while fat. Students,
although generally less sophisticated than their professional counterparts,
demonstrate a similar interest in me as an embodied fat woman, rather than
an expert on a particular topic. For instance, in a class I taught on art and
the body, we covered a variety of challenging subjects including race and

sexuality. The class openly and freely engaged in debate and the sharing of personal narratives about all topics until we reached the class on contemporary body image. That day, students expressed willingness to talk about their own personal familiarity with being discriminated against for being thin (being told to go eat a piece of pie, etc.), but exhibited reluctance to talk about any other kind of body image issue, instead asking me to share my own narrative. While this may be partially attributed to the open dialogue I encouraged in that class, the students also made it clear that they felt I was different from them and must have had different experiences or special knowledge because of my fat body. Like members of other marginalized groups, I was singled out and expected to speak as the voice of a diverse group of people sharing a particular physical characteristic.[28]

This attitude, that emotional investment compromises academic integrity, has been used to question the entire field of fat studies itself. In an article about the discipline of fat studies, Stephen H. Balch, at that time president of the National Association of Scholars, stated that "in one field after another, passion and venting have come to define the nature of what academics do. Ethnic studies, women's studies, queer studies—they're all about vindicating the grievances of some particular group. That's not what the academy should be about."[29] Beyond his egregious mischaracterization of this kind of scholarship as "venting" and "vindicating . . . grievances," Balch is reiterating in macrocosm the same idea used against individual scholars in a microcosm: that passion and intellectual rigor are mutually exclusive. This argument serves to confer particular authority on white, male scholars like Balch, who have the luxury of remaining dispassionate because they themselves do not experience the kinds of discrimination that breed intense emotion.

The privileging of one particular viewpoint as more objective and even universal has an additional consequence. Scholarship on marginalized groups becomes marginalized itself. Thus scholars writing about Native American art publish in separate journals, for instance; fat studies now has its own dedicated space in the recently established *Fat Studies: An Interdisciplinary Journal of Body Weight and Society*. While journals dedicated to particular areas of study provide useful locations for dialogue and encourage the production of knowledge for that area, it does seem that they further marginalize their topics and limit the spread of that knowledge to those already familiar with the subject matter. Should a fat-focused art historian concentrate on being published in *Fat Studies* or seek to bring her material to a wider audience, say *Art Journal* or *Art in America*? Which will look better on her CV? Which will lend her more credibility as a scholar and an expert in her field? Which will better disseminate her ideas? I don't know the answers to these questions, but I think they are important for anyone working on a topic outside of what is mainstream for his field.

BIG FAT ASSETS

Being fat presents certain challenges for scholars. It creates financial hardship and subjects you to discrimination, as in the wider world. However, being fat can be an asset in academia. Thinking back on some of the question-and-answer sessions I have participated in, I see that there is room to make this a productive space for useful dialogue. Now that I am more prepared for the kinds of personal questions that inevitably arise (and which, I would like to reiterate, no one should be expected to be asked or to answer, as no one individual is the spokesperson for his or her entire marginalized group), I think that my answers could ultimately be a way to empower myself and to bridge the gap between my understanding of the meaning of fat bodies and the audience's.

What if, when asked if I would want to pose nude, I had responded honestly about my conflicted relationship with my own body, and my fears of having such an image appropriated and used as a visual joke on the Internet—which has actually happened to more than one of the artists in my dissertation? Perhaps we could have had a meaningful conversation about the ways in which the fat body is used as a scapegoat or symbol for such disparate issues as corporate greed, prejudice and intolerance, poverty, the decline of American moral values, and so on. What if I had gently and nonaggressively turned the question around on the questioner and asked if she would feel comfortable asking that question of a thin scholar, or answering it herself? Maybe this could have started a debate about the very issues addressed in this chapter.

Finally, while being thin doesn't provide a privileged, neutral, objective viewpoint of fat bodies, and being fat doesn't provide a privileged insight into fatness, I believe that life experiences contribute to the richness of scholarship. Would the scholars I most admire write with the same nuance and empathy if they had undergone different life experiences? Could Homi K. Bhabha have so compellingly dissected Orientalism if he had been born white and in London? Could Linda Nochlin have written her seminal article, "Why Have There Been No Great Women Artists?"[30] without being a woman? Being fat has made me who I am, both as a human being and as a scholar. Had I not encountered the cognitive dissonance of being fat and yet defying the cultural stereotypes about fatness, would I have gravitated toward fat studies? My lived experience of the fat body helps me to think and write about meaningful issues, and to approach my subject matter within a more empathetic framework. So despite the fact that my fatness can negatively affect the way others perceive and receive both my body and my body of work, I consider it to be one of my biggest, fattest assets.

NOTES

1. Laura G. Knapp, Janice E. Kelly-Reid, and Scott A. Ginder, "Employees in Postsecondary Institutions, Fall 2011 and Student Financial Aid, Academic Year

2010–2011: First Look (Provisional Data)," National Center for Education Statistics, Institute of Education Sciences, U.S. Department of Education publication, September 2012, http://nces.ed.gov/pubs2012/2012156rev.pdf.

2. Anne Collins Goodyear and Linda Downs, "An Open Letter to Victoria H. F. Scott Regarding the CAA," February 8, 2013, http://www.collegeart.org/news/2013/02/08/an-open-letter-to-victoria-h-f-scott-regarding-the-caa/.

3. Thomas D. Snyder and Sally A. Dillow, "Digest of Education Statistics 2010," National Center for Education Statistics, Institute of Education Sciences, U.S. Department of Education publication, April 2011, http://nces.ed.gov/pubs2011/2011015.pdf.

4. Bill Hathaway, "Gender Bias in Hiring: Even Scientists Do It," *Fiscal Times*, September 24, 2012, http://www.thefiscaltimes.com/Articles/2012/09/24/Gender-Bias-in-Hiring-Even-Scientists-Do-It.aspx#page1.

5. Lisa Sinclair and Ziva Kunda, "Motivated Stereotyping of Women: She's Fine If She Praised Me but Incompetent If She Criticized Me," *Personality and Social Psychology Bulletin* 26, no. 11 (November 2000): 1329–42.

6. Frances Trix and Caroline Psenka, "Exploring the Color of Glass: Letters of Recommendation for Female and Male Medical Faculty," *Discourse and Society* 14, no. 2 (March 2003): 191–220.

7. Rhea E. Steinpreis, Katie A. Anders, and Dawn Ritzke, "The Impact of Gender on the Review of the Curricula Vitae of Job Applicants and Tenure Candidates: A National Empirical Study," *Sex Roles* 41, nos. 7–8 (January 1999): 509–28.

8. Ibid., 523.

9. Laurie A. Rudman and Peter Glick, "Prescriptive Gender Stereotypes and Backlash toward Agentic Women," *Journal of Social Issues* 57, no. 4 (2001): 743–62. For an excellent review of the literature on this topic, see Shelley J. Correll and Stephen Benard, "Gender and Racial Bias in Hiring," memo, March 21, 2006, http://provost.upenn.edu/uploads/media_items/gender-racial-bias.original.pdf.

10. Kerry O'Brien, as quoted in University of Manchester, "Obesity Affects Job Prospects for Women, Study Finds," *Science News*, April 30, 2012, http://www.sciencedaily.com/releases/2012/04/120430101034.htm.

11. Del Jones, "Obesity Can Mean Less Pay," *USA Today*, September 4, 2002, http://usatoday30.usatoday.com/money/workplace/2002-09-04-overweight-pay-bias_x.htm.

12. Cheryl L. Maranto and Ann Fraedrich Stenoien, "Weight Discrimination: A Multidisciplinary Analysis," *Employee Responsibilities and Rights Journal* 12, no. 1 (March 2000): 9–24; Tomas Philipson et al., "The Economics of Obesity: A Report on the Workshop Held at USDA's Economic Research Service," *Electronic Publications from the Food Assistance & Nutrition Research Program*, EFAN-04004, May 2004, n.p., http://www.ers.usda.gov/publications/efan-electronic-publications-from-the-food-assistance-nutrition-research-program/efan04004.aspx#.UaTHHlK0J8E.

13. See, for instance: M. R. Jebl and J. Xu, "Weighing the Care: Physicians' Reactions to the Size of a Patient," *International Journal of Obesity* 25, no. 8 (August 2001): 1246–52; Tara Parker-Pope, "Are Doctors Nicer to Thinner Patients?," *New York Times*, April 29, 2013, http://well.blogs.nytimes.com/2013/04/

29/overweight-patients-face-bias/; Rebecca M. Puhl and Chelsea A. Heuer, "The Stigma of Obesity: A Review and Update," *Obesity* 17, no. 5 (May 2009): 941–64, http://onlinelibrary.wiley.com/doi/10.1038/oby.2008.636/abstract; Delese Weir et al., "Making Fun of Patients: Medical Students' Perceptions and Use of Derogatory and Cynical Humor in Clinical Settings," *Academic Medicine* 81, no. 5 (May 2006): 454–62.

14. Marlene Schwartz, "Some People Would Give Life or Limb Not to Be Fat," *Yale News*, May 16, 2006, http://news.yale.edu/2006/05/16/some-people-would-give-life -or-limb-not-be-fat.

15. An Act to Prohibit Certain Food Establishments from Serving Food to Any Person Who Is Obese, Mississippi HR 282 (2008), http://billstatus.ls.state.ms.us/ 2008/pdf/history/HB/HB0282.xml. For a compact and fairly comprehensive survey of antifat bias, see also: Kelly D. Brownell et al., eds., *Weight Bias: Nature, Consequences, and Remedies* (New York: Guilford Press, 2005).

16. Being a fat student can present its own challenges, including lack of access to chairs or desks that can accommodate a person of size. For more on this topic, see Ashley Hetrick and Derek Attig, "Sitting Pretty: Fat Bodies, Classroom Desks, and Academic Excess," in *The Fat Studies Reader*, ed. Esther Rothblum and Sondra L. Solovay, 197–204 (New York: New York University Press, 2009).

17. Fat and flying is a contested issue whose implications and consequences cannot be addressed fully here. For an introduction to this troubled space from both fat-positive and antifat perspectives, see: James Durston, "Airline 'Fat Tax': Should Heavier Passengers Pay More?," CNN.com, March 26, 2013, http://travel.cnn.com/ airline-fat-tax-should-heavy-passengers-pay-more-619046; Joyce L. Huff, "Access to the Sky: Airplane Seats and Fat Bodies as Contested Spaces," in Rothblum and Solovay, *The Fat Studies Reader*, 176–86.

18. Professional appearance and conventional attractiveness matter for scholars as much as they do in the world at large. As an example, a friend of mine recently confided that during a performance evaluation at his previous (museum) job, his superior told him that he needed to start taking Rogaine if he wanted to advance in the field.

19. This term is generally used to denote those who fall somewhere between regular and plus size, so that straight-size garments are frequently too small, but plus-size garments frequently run too large; for example, a woman wearing a U.S. size 16.

20. Paul Campos, *The Obesity Myth: Why America's Obsession with Weight Is Hazardous to Your Health* (New York: Gotham Books, 2004), xxxvi, 238–45.

21. Laura Fraser, *Losing It: False Hopes and Fat Profits in the Diet Industry* (New York: Plume, 1998), 1–6.

22. Richard Klein, *Eat Fat* (New York: Pantheon, 1996), xiv–xv.

23. Marilyn Wann, *Fat!So?* (Berkeley, CA: Ten Speed Press, 1998), 9–12.

24. Shelley Bovey, *The Forbidden Body: Why Being Fat Is Not a Sin* (London: Pandora Press, 1994).

25. I should add that in all my years of attending lectures and conferences, with speakers addressing nudes from Roman to contemporary art, I have never heard another speaker get asked that question.

26. The phrasing of this idea comes directly from Melissa McEwan of *shakesville* *.com*. See her excellent posts on feminism, from which it is taken, here: Melissa McEwan, "The Terrible Bargain We Have Regretfully Struck," *Shakesville.com* (blog), August 14, 2009, http://www.shakesville.com/2009/08/terrible-bargain-we-have -regretfully.html; Melissa McEwan, "Feminism 101: 'Sexism Is a Matter of Opinion,'" *Shakesville.com* (blog), April 25, 2008, http://www.shakesville.com/2008/04/feminism -101-sexism-is-matter-of.html.

27. Kyriarchy is a term coined by scholar Elisabeth Schüssler Fiorenza to describe interconnected and interacting systems of domination in which a person may be privileged in some relationships while still being oppressed in others; in other words, a gay white man may still be privileged via his race and gender while being discriminated against for his sexuality. Kyriarchy includes sexism, racism, classism, and other forms of internalized and institutionalized hierarchy.

28. For an interesting look at the teaching of fat studies while being fat, see Elena Andrea Escalera, "Stigma Threat and the Fat Professor: Reducing Student Prejudice in the Classroom," in Rothblum and Solovay, *The Fat Studies Reader*, 205–12.

29. As quoted in Abby Ellin, "Big People on Campus," *New York Times*, November 26, 2006, http://www.nytimes.com/2006/11/26/fashion/26fat.html? pagewanted=all.

30. Linda Nochlin, "Why Have There Been No Great Women Artists?," *Art News* 69 (January 1971): 22–39.

15

Never Delivering the Whole Package: Family Influence on Fat Daughters' College Experiences

Heather Brown

When I started my research into the experiences of fat women learners at a small liberal arts college (SLAC) in the Midwest, I expected to hear many tales of doom and gloom, of teasing by classmates and overt discrimination by professors. As a fat woman learner who had recently returned to the classroom, I had experienced these things myself. My experiences as a student reinforced what I was reading in the literature —at least in the literature that was willing to explore the connections between weight discrimination and academic achievement rather than blaming the size of fat learners—and their size alone—for any challenges they might experience in school.

I did not expect to find a clear and compelling picture of how families overwhelmingly influenced their fat daughters' college experiences and their understandings of themselves as competent learners. Indeed, these women identified their parents as the most important influence in their understanding of themselves as valuable, worthwhile, and capable learners, as young women who could do anything, learn anything, and go out and make a difference in the world. When that support was positive or neutral, fat women learners viewed themselves as capable of meeting their educational goals, including enrolling in college, as any other student. When their families focused on the size of their bodies persistently and negatively, these fat, young women felt like failures, no matter how well they did as students. Many of the women I interviewed experienced both influences from their families, leaving them confused about how the families that supported them so strongly in their pursuit of education could be so unsupportive and even cruel about the size of their bodies. They experienced the power of size privilege, which dictates that no matter their successes as students, fat women learners can never "deliver the whole package"—a package that has brains, talent, and service to others, and is also thin.

OVERVIEW OF STUDY

What little research has been done on the experiences of fat learners has focused on students from prekindergarten to high school. Almost no effort has been made to understand the experiences of fat women learners in the college environment. Instead, most research has used economic, sociological, or medical theories to speculate as to why fat female learners often exhibit poor academic achievement.

I wanted to ask different questions. I wanted to know how fat women learners perceived their own experiences as learners at the college level. To explore this question, I undertook a basic, interpretive qualitative study. Qualitative studies are "systemic, empirical strateg[ies] for answering questions about people in a particular social context" and provide "a means for describing and attempting to understand the observed regularities in what people do, or in what they report as their experiences."[1] Qualitative research methods guided by a critical fat studies perspective grounded in feminist theory have proven particularly fruitful for the type of questions I wanted to explore because they allowed me to uncover "previously silenced or forgotten experiences" of fat women learners.[2]

I conducted a series of semistructured interviews with 13 undergraduate women students who wore women's size 12 and above and were currently enrolled at SLACs. The median clothing size of the group was 18, while the mean age was 20. Among participants, seven identified as sophomores in the fall semester of 2011–12, while six identified as seniors. Juniors were unrepresented in the group, possibly because juniors are the group at SLACs most likely to study off-campus in the fall. I did not actively seek out first-year students for participation in this study because they would have had less than one semester's experience on campus at the time of the interviews. Moreover, no first-year students volunteered to participate.

Participants came from a wide range of socioeconomic backgrounds. Two self-identified as coming from upper-income families, six as middle-class, three as working-class, and two as coming from impoverished families living in inner-city areas. In terms of racial/ethnic self-identification, seven participants identified as white, four as Latina, and two as African American. No one self-identified as disabled, although two participants did self-identify as having mental health issues including situational depression and bipolar affective disorder. Eight participants identified as first-generation college students, much higher than the percentage of first-generation students in the overall population at SLACs.

GOING TO COLLEGE

The literature on fat women learners portrays them as facing significant barriers and challenges to academic success that other learners do not face. Fat women are not as likely as nonfat women to pursue postsecondary education even when they are intellectually capable and want to do so.[3] Fat women have been found to have low aspiration to attend college, a problem that has grown more prevalent in recent years.[4] Some researchers argue that fat women learners from Asian American, Hispanic, and Caucasian backgrounds are less likely to complete high school on time or enroll in and complete college,[5] while others suggest that fat adolescents in the United States are different from nonfat adolescents not only educationally but also psychologically and socially.[6] Specifically, fat female learners are far more likely to be held back a grade and to perceive themselves as poor students. Some of this literature presents these barriers and challenges to success as originating in the student herself, rather than originating in a specific situation or a social context, such as transitioning to college. For example, according to Joseph J. Sabia, the strong correlation between poor academic achievement and weight is a result of a shared lack of discipline.[7] Sabia speculates that "the least disciplined individuals are most likely to become obese and to achieve less in school."[8] In other words, fat individuals do not invest in their physical appearance and/or health and, in addition, do not invest in their educations because they are undisciplined and lazy.

However, all of the participants in my study had completed high school on time and were expecting to complete college, even though a few of them did struggle with academic achievement levels that might prevent them from graduating within four years. In addition, participants in this study, if they were struggling to succeed academically in college, attributed this struggle not to their weight but to other problems that all "normal" college students experience.

What does it mean to be a "normal" college student? I did not set out to find the answer to that question or even to compare and contrast the lives of fat women learners with the lives of students who were not fat. However, participants in this study spent a significant amount of time discussing their lives as college students, apologizing for not having "anything interesting" to tell me, and asserting that they were not any different than any other student on campus. They insisted that they struggled with the same challenges their nonfat peers did. For example, the fat women learners who participated in my study complained that their parents could not always help them navigate sometimes overwhelming obstacles.

Several participants struggled with a lack of parental moral and emotional support as well as the inability of their families to provide practical, useful advice. In most cases, the lack of support was more a form of benign neglect born out of a lack of understanding about what it means to be a college student rather than an active attempt to undermine a child's academic success. This was particularly the case among those study participants who were first-generation college students, especially when their families did not encourage them to pursue postsecondary education. For example, Tisha's family did not actively promote the pursuit of postsecondary education in their children, although her father, an older man who had completed only the seventh grade, was supportive when Tisha indicated that she was most definitely going to submit applications. In a conversation they had only a few months before he passed away, she said, "I remember before he died, he was like 'Do you plan on going to college?' and I'm like 'Yeah, of course,' and he's like 'Okay, that's good.' Me and my mom didn't really talk about it at all." The push for her to attend college came from her school. Her inner-city high school required her to apply to a certain number of colleges in order to graduate.

For other first-generation college students in my study, the expectation that they would attend and complete postsecondary education was there, even if the practical support needed to thrive in college was not always available. The manifestation of that expectation took very different forms in each young woman's family. In some cases, the young woman's family actively promoted her pursuit of a college education. In others, that expectation came from the young woman's own desire to have a better life.

Ann's family expected her to attend college, and while they did not discuss this expectation with her either, when it came time for Ann to start thinking about her educational future, her mother took an active role. Ann remembers being far more tranquil about her educational future than her mother was. Her mother actually went out and gathered application materials and filled them out for Ann. In Ann's case, her mother's active role in getting Ann to college stemmed from concerns that Ann was "too relaxed." "She had doubts, as well, I mean, 'cuz I was just a relaxed high schooler. I got the grades without doing a lot, and she was kind of worried for me, but she didn't want to see me not go. She knew that wasn't an option." Ann actually perceived her family's support of her as putative pressure rather than support. "It's not like they know this is something I've really been wanting to do and they want to see me succeed and if I wanted to drop out right now and move to New York to be a fashion designer, they'd support me? No." For Ann, the importance of education and the expectation that she would get an education has remained of critical importance to her family.

Kari's mother actively promoted college to her daughter because it was an opportunity she herself had not had. "My mom has always wanted me to get a better education since she didn't get to, so she actually started looking at colleges my junior year." Kari wondered if her mother was beginning the search too early, but her mother told her that starting the search and finding the right place was of paramount importance. "She started talking to me about college, and she's like, 'I think you're going to find a place where you're going to fit in and you'll feel so much better.'" Finding the place where her daughter could not only get a good education but enjoy the experience and grow as a person was important to her.

SUPPORTING FAT DAUGHTERS AS COLLEGE STUDENTS

Among the young women in my study, weight played little part in parental expectations that their fat daughters would or would not pursue postsecondary education. In most cases, college was the path they were expected to take after graduating from high school, either because it was what their parents wanted or because it was what the women themselves felt they should do, and, therefore, it was the path they pursued. They also perceived that they received a significant amount of support from their families as they enrolled in college and as they worked toward earning their degrees.

Financial support from their family was the type of support most mentioned by participants in my study. Betsy earned a scholarship to attend college, but it did not cover the entire cost. Her family paid for everything not covered by her scholarship. This financial support was one of the keys to Betsy's success in school. "I don't know what I would do if I had to pay for it all on my own. I think that would put a lot of pressure on me, and I wouldn't be able to work as hard as I can, 'cuz I'd have that and I wouldn't be supported by my parents and then I wouldn't feel like I was doing my best at school." Betsy's mother also provided her with the moral support and encouragement that she needed to help her stay in school when an overwhelming semester nearly led her to quit:

> Last year, I was really stressed out because I had a final paper due in every class and then a final exam in a couple of classes, and I told my mom I didn't want to finish. It was too hard. I couldn't handle it, and she told me that in order to do that I would have to drop out and then she said that I worked too hard for that, and it wasn't worth it, so I was like, oh okay, yeah, I'll try and see what this is like. I ended up doing okay on all that, actually doing great on some of them, so that made me realize I could do this. I can do college. It's not as bad as I thought it was, and I could do another whole year of it, and now I don't have those feelings at all. I don't want to drop out. I really want to finish.

By helping Betsy make it through a difficult stage of her academic journey, Betsy's mother helped her develop a strong sense of her ability to accomplish even the most difficult of learning tasks.

Family support also helped many of the participants in my study develop a healthy self-esteem and a deeply ingrained understanding that they are capable of accomplishing their tasks and meeting their goals. For example, Stacy credits her mother for helping her develop a strong self-esteem and for encouraging her to be successful, even though she is not perfect. "I feel like I have very good self-esteem. I definitely got that from my mom. She's always tried to teach me to be the best that I can." Her mother also encouraged her to develop independence and to trust herself. "Trying to be independent also has given me that edge of self-confidence that you can depend on other people but it really truly matters what you think of yourself and what you think of the things you're doing." Juanita's parents encouraged her to be the best she can be. "They're always telling me to do my best. They always say 'try,' 'cuz it takes a lot of hard work, but it's gonna be worth it in the end."

The young women in my study received the financial support of their families to the best of their families' abilities to provide it. This presents a more nuanced picture of previous research, which found that families are less likely to pay tuition for their fat daughters' educations, forcing them to seek employment and student loans, whereas these same families paid for their fat sons' educations.[9] Crandall also found that fat daughters were more likely to have to work or take out student loans than other learners, putting them at a major disadvantage in completing their education and performing well academically.[10] Participants in my study took advantage of all the financial support options available to them and also received the financial support of their parents when it was possible for families to provide that support. Families supported their daughters financially whenever possible, regardless of their daughters' weight.

FAT IS FAILURE, BODY AND MIND

Families with fat daughters were promotive of their daughters' educational aspirations and provided a significant amount of moral and financial support. However, fat female learners reported a significant amount of contention between themselves and their families in regard to their body weight. They perceived that they are on the receiving end of a significant amount of "fat talk" from their families, particularly the distaff sides of their families. Fat talk is talk revolving around issues of dieting and grounded in constant references to weight, even and especially when what the individual wants to discuss has nothing to do with weight and everything to do with issues of power and control.[11] The young women in my study reported that their mothers dieted with them or pressured them to pursue dieting. While much of the diet talk was couched in terms of health concerns and was perceived by study participants as coming from a place of genuine care, some families teased or bullied their fat daughters about their weight. No matter the impetus for the body disparagement, it led these young women to question their self-worth. Because they were fat, they were, many perceived, somehow defective or less capable. Not only did dieting and fat talk affect their self-image; in some cases, it affected or continues to affect their academic performance.

When asked who affected their perceptions of themselves as learners the most, the fat female learners in my study told me that their families did. Friends can be changed, but family is forever. Many participants spoke highly of their families, especially about their families' encouragement of them to pursue a college education as well as the financial support they provided. In a few cases, participants also spoke about how their families worked to build their self-esteem, particularly their body image. For example, Mercedes never understood how larger women could have poor body image or low self-esteem because her family encouraged her to love her large body. Her mother "used to put me in front of the mirror and say 'Oh, look at you. You're so beautiful' and just reinforce our self-esteem and now she calls me a monster because I just love myself so much. I'd be like I can love myself or I can have low self-esteem. You pick one!" Mercedes credits her mother with helping her develop the self-esteem she needed to thrive in a boarding school and then in college.

Unfortunately, most of the study participants experienced the opposite from their families. Rather than being told they are beautiful and having their families help them develop a positive body image, most of them experienced significant pressure from their families to diet and lose weight. This pressure most often came from their mothers, who would try to spur weight loss in their fat daughters by dieting with them.

For example, Amanda's battles with her mother about weight began in junior high school. At the age of 12, she and her mother spent a summer doing a low-carbohydrate diet, and while her mother lost and kept off a significant amount of weight, Amanda did not. Amanda's lack of weight loss became a major issue between the two. During her freshman year of high school, Amanda's mother would weigh her every morning. If Amanda had gained weight, she was not allowed to spend time with friends or would lose her allowance, making her feel even worse about herself. As she felt worse about herself, she often overate, leading to additional weight gain. The stress of the situation also began to affect her grades. These battles continued even though Amanda separated herself from her family by going to a different continent to attend college.

As she continued college, however, things improved for Amanda. "It just continued to get better and better each semester. My grades got better. I mean they never were bad, but I just sort of got more and more into [SLAC]. I sort of found my place, and I loved my girlfriend, and just things, you know, just got better, and now I think they're the best they've ever been."

Her relationship with her mother also improved. Amanda, during her four years of college, developed an understanding of her mother's behavior and developed a sort of peace with her. "I don't think she ever did anything just to be mean, but she had been overweight, and she wanted this so badly for me. She wanted me to have everything."

The relationship between families and their fat daughters is often challenging, particularly if the family wishes the fat daughter to lose weight. One question this research sought to explore was whether or not fat women learners perceived that they were the target of weight-based discrimination by members of their families and, if so, what effect this bias had on their experiences as learners. For most of the participants in my study, their families told them over and over again, at various levels of compassion or derision, that they were fat and that being fat was problematic. Just as Carla Rice found in her study, the participants in this study developed an identity centered on their weight early in their lives and that identity as a weighted body affected the young women's sense of themselves as college students.[12] Their formation of the self as a fat body in a culture that devalues and disparages the fat body caused participants to struggle with the development and maintenance of positive body image and self-esteem because their bodies were devalued. Many of them also struggled with depression.

Study participants who were on the receiving end of fat talk from family members or were pressured by their families to lose weight all commented on how damaging it was to their self-esteem. For example, as a result of the fighting between herself and her mother about weight, Amanda, in the early years of her college career, felt like a failure, like someone who "could just never deliver the whole package," the whole package being one that had all of Amanda's skills and talents but was wrapped in a slender body.

Kari perceived that the harassment she received from her family about her weight undercut her faith in her intellectual abilities. After talking about how her grandmother had constantly belittled her about her weight and, at one point, offered to pay her for every pound she could lose, she said:

> I think for a long time, weight was part of the reason why I didn't think I could get into college, which of course has nothing to do with it. But I think I had that tendency of, like, I'm not good enough, and that was the main reason. It's not necessarily that I wasn't smart enough or I didn't have the grades, or I didn't have the extra-curriculars or I don't have the resume or whatever to get in. It was just the idea that I'm not good enough, and it was because I'm fat. I'm just not gonna be able to do it.

While Kari was able to fight back against feelings of unworthiness triggered in her by her family's disparagement of her body, Ann learned to project a fake image of herself as a confident, competent learner to those around her. This self-confidence is all an act, she feels, because any chance she had at developing a true sense of deep-seated self-confidence was destroyed by years of body disparagement she received from her family. "I was told by my mother my whole life to love and accept myself, but you need, you should probably go on a diet. So I don't [have good self-esteem]. I fake it." She described these messages as particularly hurtful because they came from her family: "That can be hurtful, especially coming from someone being so critical. This is your home. This is your family."

Poor self-esteem, depression, and a lack of understanding about why her weight was so much more important than anything else in her life to her family also plagued Elmira. Her family harassed her about her weight every time she visited them. "Every time I'm there, it's like how you should lose weight or aren't you unhappy with the way you are? You know, I'm not gonna say I'm 100% happy with who I am, but I've grown accustomed to it. I don't really expect more, because I'm so focused on other things. It's like for me weight is no longer the biggest issue. I have more important things to worry about." Doing well in college was one of those concerns.

Coming to this realization required Elmira to overcome a lifetime of mocking about her weight, but her journey is not over. Despite her brave talk and the great strides she has made in building her self-confidence and a positive image of herself as a successful learner, the body disparagement directed at her by her family has resulted in lingering scars as well as confusion about why, like Amanda's parents, Elmira's parents cannot accept her as the whole package:

> When I was younger, they used to make a lot of jokes at my expense and call me names and say really, really horrible things that to them was funny. I didn't say anything. I was always that really quiet child, but I guess that stuff sort of stuck with me. It was kind of hard, I mean in high school, because I was away. I missed my family, but I still had that sort of resentment towards them, and then sort of resentment towards myself because I sort of let myself become so overweight. That caused me to be depressed.

This weight-related depression is something she struggled with throughout her college career. She also found it hard to reconcile the support they had given her as a student with the harassment they had given her about her weight.

Robert Crosnoe and Chandra Muller suggest that fat female learners are aware that others around them judge them as deficient because they are fat.[13] As a result of this awareness, they develop a poor self-concept and exhibit "hamper[ed] adjustment and functioning."[14] These consequences of being judged in this way are especially visible in an environment, such as college, where there is a conflict between the student's existence as a fat body and an environment where thinness is excessively valued.[15]

Study participants' experiences suggest that the environment in which they developed an understanding of themselves as deficient because of their bodies was not school but rather the home. Home, in nearly every participant's case, was the setting in which they experienced the most consistent and virulent body disparagement, pressure to diet, and exposure to fat talk. The family that wants their fat daughter to be thin constitutes a threatening environment

According to Michael Inzlicht and Catherine Good, threatening environments are those "where people come to suspect that they could be devalued, stigmatized, or discriminated against because of a particular social identity."[16] The result of being exposed to a threatening environment is that the environment lowers the exposed individual's self-concept and self-esteem, often leading to lowered academic achievement and a negative self-esteem that infiltrates every aspect of life.

For study participants, the family was and, for some, continued to be a threatening environment. Their families either suggested they lose weight or teased and mocked them about their weight. Even those who have lived away from home for several years were subjected to this behavior during visits. Because they were heavy and their families made them aware that this is not how they were supposed to be, many of these young women felt that despite getting good grades, staying out of trouble, and working hard, they were never quite good enough for their families. As college students, they still struggled with feeling not quite good enough to succeed.

For Mercedes self-esteem, and not a thin body, is the key to academic success:

> It's sad that weight issues have been a deterrent for some people with their education because, like I said, it has nothing to do with your abilities, but again, I think that family support also has a little pull in that. If you don't have your support from your family, then weight is just another thing that the world is telling you is wrong with you, and it's just another thing to discourage you even if it's not the reason your family doesn't support you. It just becomes an additional struggle. Nobody should really have to do that and deal with that.

Unfortunately, many fat female learners at the college level do have to deal with disparagement from their families. They've had to deal with it from the time they were young girls. As a result, many of them struggle with depression, low self-esteem, and poor body image. These struggles have affected their academic performance and their sense of themselves as capable learners. The literature that exists on the academic achievement of fat women learners at the postsecondary level does not address the impact of family disparagement on the outcomes of this population; my data suggest that the family might play a significant role in the success and failure of their fat daughters as undergraduate learners.

WHAT IT ALL MEANS: THE POWER OF SIZE PRIVILEGE

Samantha Kwan discusses "body privilege" as "an invisible package of unearned assets that thin or normal-sized individuals can take for granted on a daily basis."[17] I expand on Kwan's concept by calling it size privilege. This term serves to further delineate that the concept is specifically addressing the unearned privileges associated with being or aspiring to be an (ever-changing) culturally "ideal" body size, currently a particular level of thinness, particularly among women. Using the term "size privilege," I suggest, allows for a differentiation between the privileges associated with so-called ideal weight as opposed to unearned privileges associated with other bodily states of being, such as able-bodiedness. Using the term "size privilege" acknowledges that although we believe that individuals of a certain "ideal" weight possess privilege in Western culture, even those who are at that "ideal" weight must still struggle with their bodies in order to maintain that privilege, which is not only elusive but often temporary as the definition of "ideal" weight constantly evolves. The concept of size privilege also challenges Kwan's use of the term "normal-sized" in her definition. Using the term "normal-sized" is in and of itself an exercise of "body privilege" because it axiomatically defines the fat body as non-normative and stigmatizes it even while trying to point out how the privilege associated with thin bodies is unearned and problematic.

Size privilege is not necessarily a new concept, however. That thinness is privileged and fatness considered immoral, sick, and deviant in modern Western culture and that women bear the brunt of responsibility for maintaining their bodies in a state of slenderness (an ever-changing and unreachable goal) is not a new theory; it has been identified in numerous feminist writings since at least the 1970s.[18]

In the critical fat studies literature, the ideas inherent in size privilege have been expressed in multiple ways. For example, Laura Fraser describes the "inner corset."[19] Based on the Victorian practice of shaping the female body into a specific culturally ideal shape through the use of restrictive and dangerous corsets, the inner corset represents the powerful cultural forces that keep women in the Western world "preoccupied with slenderness and with the project of losing weight at all costs."[20] This preoccupation with slenderness could not happen if women did not, at least at some level, understand the power and privilege associated with the "ideal" body and fear the consequences of not being or of not striving to be that "ideal" body. According to Fraser:

> We still live with the Victorian myth that all of us, no matter what our shape, build, or age, should be able to fit on a single scale of ideal weights, and that if we tip the scale, we have only ourselves to blame. Most of us don't recognize that the social forces that keep pulling us toward thinness are every bit as constraining as the corsets that kept our great-great-grandmothers from actively participating in the world. Nor do we realize that the inner corset we wear is one of the strongest and most insidious remnants of oppression against women that we still put up with. Instead, we hate our feminine bodies—which naturally have more fat than men's, allowing us to bear and nurse children and survive during times of famine—and blame ourselves for not controlling them. We don't imagine that real freedom, choice, and respect for ourselves would mean accepting our bodies the way they are.[21]

In recent writings, the characteristics of size privilege are most often discussed through the lens of bias and discrimination, focusing on the consequences that fat women face in a fat-hating world. Nita Mary McKinley suggests that discussions of weight are nearly always political and that the political nature of these discussions "highlights the use of fatness as a status variable through which certain groups of people can be stigmatized and exploited."[22] Janna L. Fikkan and Esther D. Rothblum further argue that thinness as a privileged cultural ideal is detrimental for nearly all women because the privileging of thinness and the devaluing of fatness lead to significant life-altering discrimination, particularly for women.[23] "It is not enough to note that the ever thinner cultural ideal means that practically every woman will feel badly about her body. Feminists also need to turn our collective attention to the reality that, because of the pervasiveness and gendered nature of weight-based stigma, a majority of women stand to *suffer significant discrimination* because they do not conform to this ever-narrower standard."[24]

CONCLUSION

Marilyn Wann suggests that everyone is touched and influenced by weight bias; weight bias is a direct consequence of size privilege.[25] The effects of body disparagement by family members showed the power of size privilege in the college experiences of study participants. Participants did not wholeheartedly agreed with family statements about the inappropriateness of their fat bodies nor could they easily reconcile their families' obvious and significant support of them as college students with their families' obvious and significant "concern" about their fat bodies. In these situations, participants' reactions to size privilege and to being treated poorly because they lack this privilege manifested in feelings of confusion, sadness, and failure. As families insisted that their fat daughters lose weight, many study participants felt the full brunt of size privilege. Because they were fat bodies, they could never be quite good enough. There was always something wrong with them, even if they succeeded in every other area of their life. Nothing else about them mattered— not good grades and not success in every other area of life. Despite encouragement to attend college, despite financial and other forms of support from their families once they enrolled, fat female students are not able to deliver the complete (thin) package their families expected.

NOTES

1. Lawrence F. Locke, Waneen Wyrick Spirduso, and Stephen J. Silverman, *Proposals That Work: A Guide for Planning Dissertations and Grant Proposals* (Thousand Oaks, CA: Sage, 2007), 96.

2. Abigail Brooks and Sharlene Nagy Hesse-Biber, "An Invitation to Feminist Research," in *Feminist Research Practice: A Primer*, ed. Sharlene Nagy Hesse-Biber and Patricia Lina Leavy (Thousand Oaks, CA: Sage, 2007), 11.

3. Helen Canning and Jean Mayer, "Obesity—Its Possible Effect on College Acceptance," *New England Journal of Medicine* 275, no. 21 (1966): 1172–74; Helen Canning and Jean Mayer, "Obesity: An Influence on High School Performance?," *The American Journal of Clinical Nutrition* 20, no. 4 (1967): 352–54; Robert Crosnoe, "Gender, Obesity, and Education," *Sociology of Education* 80, no. 3 (2007): 241–60.

4. Kylie Ball, David Crawford, and Justin Kenardy, "Longitudinal Relationships among Overweight, Life Satisfaction, and Aspirations in Young Women," *Obesity Research* 12, no. 6 (2004): 1019–30; Angela G. Fowler-Brown et al., "Adolescent Obesity and Future College Degree Attainment," *Obesity* 18, no. 6 (2009): 1235–41.

5. Albert A. Okunade, Andrew J. Hussey, and Mustafa C. Karakus, "Overweight Adolescents and On-Time High School Graduation: Racial and Gender Disparities," *Atlantic Economic Journal* 37, no. 3 (2009): 225–42.

6. Nicole H. Falkner et al., "Social, Educational, and Psychological Correlates of Weight Status in Adolescents," *Obesity Research* 9, no. 1 (2001): 32–42.

7. Joseph J. Sabia, "The Effect of Body Weight on Adolescent Academic Performance," *Southern Economic Journal* 73, no. 4 (2007): 871–900.

8. Ibid., 873.

9. Christian S. Crandall, "Do Heavy-Weight Students Have More Difficulty Paying for College?," *Personality and Social Psychology Bulletin* 17, no. 6 (1991): 606–11; Christian S. Crandall, "Do Parents Discriminate against Their Heavyweight Daughters?," *Personality and Social Psychology Bulletin* 21, no. 7 (1995): 724–35.

10. Crandall, "Do Heavy-Weight Students"; Crandall, "Do Parents Discriminate."

11. Mimi Nichter, *Fat Talk: What Girls and Their Parents Say about Dieting* (Cambridge, MA: Harvard University Press, 2009).

12. Carla Rice, "Becoming 'The Fat Girl': Acquisition of an Unfit Identity," *Women's Studies International Forum* 30, no. 2 (2007): 158–74.

13. Robert Crosnoe and Chandra Muller, "Body Mass Index, Academic Achievement, and School Context: Examining the Educational Experiences of Adolescents at Risk of Obesity," *Journal of Health and Social Behavior* 45, no. 4 (2004): 393–407.

14. Ibid., 394.

15. Crosnoe and Muller, "Body Mass Index"; Dana Heller Levitt, "Drive for Thinness and Fear of Fat among College Women: Implications for Practice and Assessment," *Journal of College Counseling* 7, no. 2 (2004): 109–17.

16. Michael Inzlicht and Catherine Good, "How Environments Can Threaten Academic Performance, Self-Knowledge, and Sense of Belonging," in *Stigma and Group Inequality: Social Psychological Perspectives*, ed. Shana Levin and Colette van Laar (Mahwah, NJ: Erlbaum, 2006), 131.

17. Samantha Kwan, "Navigating Public Spaces: Gender, Race, and Body Privilege in Everyday Life," *Feminist Formations* 22, no. 2 (2010): 147.

18. Janna L. Fikkan and Esther D. Rothblum, "Is Fat a Feminist Issue? Exploring the Gendered Nature of Weight Bias," *Sex Roles* 66, nos. 9–10 (2012): 575–92.

19. Laura Fraser, *Losing It: America's Obsession with Weight and the Industry That Feeds on It* (New York: Dutton, 1997).

20. Ibid., 282.

21. Ibid.

22. Nita Mary McKinley, "Ideal Weight/Ideal Women," in *Weighty Issues: Fatness and Thinness as Social Problems*, ed. Jeffery Sobal and Donna Maurer (New York: Aldine de Gruyter, 1999), 109.

23. Fikkan and Rothblum, "Is Fat a Feminist Issue?"

24. Ibid., 578.

25. Marilyn Wann, "Fat Studies: An Invitation to Revolution," in *The Fat Studies Reader*, ed. Esther D. Rothblum and Sondra Solovay (New York: New York University Press, 2009), xxi–xxv.

16

The University: 10 Lessons about Health Promotions from a Big 10 University

Ronda Bokram

For the past 25 years I have been a staff nutritionist with the Health Education Department of Olin, the student health center at Michigan State University. By education and training, I am a registered dietitian who graduated with a BS in clinical dietetics from Michigan State University in 1977 and a Master's in nutrition from the University of Wisconsin in 1980. I was trained to give low-calorie (1,200–1,500) diets to individuals who wanted to lose weight. I would "knowledgably" tell people what they "should" and "should not" eat to be "healthy." There were rules for all aspects of nutrition that I learned and would espouse with the goal always of helping people. It seemed so clear what I needed to do, was supposed to do, and should do. Never in my training or education was I taught to consider how people felt or thought or how those aspects impacted what they actually did or felt about themselves. I wasn't even taught this in regard to working with an individual struggling with an eating disorder. As I observed weight loss failure after failure, I knew I could not continue to recommend an approach that was doomed to failure in terms of long-term weight loss (or any at all for that matter), created problems for an individual psychologically, and as I later learned, had no scientific basis for recommending. I knew there must be another way, another approach, but what?

Luckily, during my first year at Michigan State University (1988), Jane Hirshman and Carol Munter recognized the connection between restrictive eating and the tendency to "inhale" food later. They developed an approach to working with individuals and groups that was published in the book titled *Overcoming Overeating: How to Break the Diet/Binge Cycle and Live a Healthier, More Satisfying Life*. Other books, such as *Breaking Free from Emotional Eating* (2004) by Geneen Roth and *Intuitive Eating* (2003) by Evelyn Tribole and Elyse Resch, were published. They all encouraged taking the focus from external control of what one ate to working with one's internal cues of hunger, appetite, and satiety, acknowledging the impact of one's emotional relationship with eating, and learning how to trust oneself around food and eating. These nondieting approaches made sense and make sense still. I started to change how I approach nutrition with the students I worked with and continue to work with at the university. I began to see not only that diets do not work in the long run but that the psychological impact of feeling that "you" (the dieter) are the problem (not the diet) is significant; I began to see how this creates self-blame for failing at the diet ("I just didn't do it well enough"), body loathing (especially if you lost some weight but then gained it back, or couldn't lose any at all), and ultimately low self-esteem. And, even as significantly, that weight loss did not guarantee better health.

Professional ignorance and an academically learned narrow approach to health and nutrition are my rationale (excuse) for how I approached nutrition with the students I interacted with initially. I now know more, know better, and for many years have had the opportunity (and the challenge) to do nutrition education, counseling, and activism in a way and with an approach that makes sense professionally and personally. As I reflect on the past 25 years, and in consideration of writing this chapter, I can certainly categorize key factors and concepts that I have had to address in my work as a dietitian at Michigan State—factors that have been barriers as well as assets in the work I do in attempting to create positive changes and truly focus on health for both individuals and the university community.

UNDERSTANDING HOW PEOPLE THINK IS CRITICAL

Another way to say this is the "why" of what people believe or feel impacts the "what" of the behaviors in which they tend to engage. I often feel that I should have gotten a degree in psychology rather than nutrition. I might then have been ahead of the game instead of in the "learn as I go" track. Truly, this has been absolutely critical in the work that I do. Knowledge is rational, logical, often concrete, but feelings are so much more powerful. Peers, family, media, and individual experiences all significantly contribute to how we feel about ourselves, others, and around body image; and that can determine your relationship with food and ultimately yourself.

Most of the students I have worked with have had nutrition in their health classes during high school, or they have taken a nutrition class at Michigan State. They know how to read labels; they know there is a recommended daily intake of nutrients that they require. They will ignore all of that, eat much less then they need—eliminate food that would promote bone density, for example—if they believe it means they will weigh less or have the opportunity to change their body shape or size. You truly cannot help individuals with nutrition for their health until you understand their relationship with food and their body. It is so important to take time to understand them as people, to get beneath the surface and understand how they think in order to help them see themselves as not just a number on a scale or body mass index (BMI) chart. *Only then* can you work with them to look at their sense of self and their nutrition in a manner that truly will benefit their health, both physiologically and psychologically, for the rest of their lives.

When students do begin to recognize this, it is almost as if a burden has been taken off their shoulders. It is freeing in many ways. They can actually spend time thinking of other aspects of their lives instead of calculating what they should and should not have, feeling like failures when they can't or don't lose weight, failures when they gain it back, always blaming themselves rather than the weight loss attempt or focus. I am very fortunate to have this time with each student that I work with, though they do not all embrace this different approach. But I always say, each interaction is an opportunity to provide an approach to these areas that they have never heard before and might not be ready to hear now. When they are ready, they may remember what I said or come back to revisit and make changes. This has happened many times, and I have learned to be patient, as internal change takes longer but can last forever.

SCIENCE IS NOT NECESSARILY AN ALLY

We need science. Good research helps reaffirm what we believe, open our eyes to new ideas and products, and provide support for what we, as professionals, teach to those with whom we interact. Science is important. Unfortunately, the literal following of science in terms of nutrition guidelines (i.e., calories, milligrams, grams, etc.) leads individuals to a very rigid approach to eating. I keep a box of Pop-Tarts in my office. I like Pop-Tarts; I rediscovered them when I had children, and I do not consider them a "bad food." I keep that box there as many of the students who I interact with do consider them a "bad" food. (I even had a dietitian tell me once that they were toxic.) When I ask a student why they are "bad," they usually respond with something about the carbohydrate content, the sugar content, not enough protein, too many calories, or a combination of those. I respond by saying that this might be a problem if all I ate was Pop-Tarts, but if I eat Pop-Tarts along with other foods, does it really have that much of an impact one way or another? After all, isn't nutrition really about how we eat over time? And should any food have the ability to make you feel guilty, feel "fat," feel bad about yourself? It is just food, not good or bad, just food.

It is important to use nutrition science to create an inclusive, not exclusive, approach to eating. When individuals are using a food label to restrict, they are giving it the power to tell them whether they are okay or not, and that is a lot of power to give to any food. There is no one way to eat that will cause you to lose weight, gain weight, stay the same, never get cancer, get cancer, and I could go on and on. The research provides general guidelines, not individualized advice. If you are in this field long enough, you also know that science and recommendations can change. However, your genetics, and who and where you came from, do not and cannot be changed. As I tell the students, we keep science in mind, but let's be open to an approach that will help you achieve health in a manner that is enhancing rather than restrictive, that isn't focused on your BMI or weight, and that teaches you to work with your specific needs and potential, and builds a positive sense of self and body image. That is within you, not in a scientific journal or book at the library.

THE DOWNSIDE OF TECHNOLOGY

I sometimes wish that apps and other electronic advancements would just not be so available. Understand, I was initially a computer science major; I even worked at a computer center at Dow Chemical in Midland, Michigan, where I grew up. Computers are amazing, especially for traveling or communicating with others around the world. However, the apps that have become so readily accessible to students for calculating calories in food portions, setting weight loss goals, and calculating calories burned have become a nemesis to those of us trying to promote positive eating and healthy relationships with food and body image.

In the past you had to read an article on how to lose weight and get the summer "beach body." Now you can now calculate every calorie you eat, check your intake throughout the day, ask your iPhone if you can eat anymore during the day or have eaten too much (and then, of course, feel bad about yourself either way)—all in the palm of your hand. These apps externalize everything about your relationship with food. They are the same as diets, providing external control that can turn into rigid patterns and lead to failure and another diet, or increasingly disordered eating.

Another downside to technology are the numerous, truly uncountable websites that promote dieting, thinness, and even eating disorders. It is common knowledge that almost every commercial photo is digitally altered, and yet that knowledge doesn't stop these images from creating an unattainable stereotype of beauty. They are still powerful motivators for comparison and body loathing among vulnerable students.

As I try to help people learn to develop trust within themselves, to give themselves permission to eat, to develop positive relationships with food and their body, these have proven to be powerful and unfortunate tools in promoting exactly the opposite.

This easy access to superficial information and limited ability or willingness to critique what they see and read, to question what they are hearing or seeing, can and does have enormous psychological impact for individuals. In fact, one of the most common statements I hear in my office is "But 'they' say . . ." When I ask who "they" is, the usual response is "You know, they." What usually comes out is that "they" is someone or something they heard on television, read in the news, or found online. It could have even been an infomercial or advertisement on Facebook. At no point was the credibility of "they" checked out. But because what "they" say is commonly heard or believed, it is accepted as truth when it could be the furthest thing from it. In an effort to counter "they," I have developed a lending library of appropriate and truly helpful books and videos that students can borrow. It allows students more opportunity to consider their approaches to food, their body, and their health to be challenged outside my office as they were within my office.

RECYCLING IS GREAT FOR THE ENVIRONMENT BUT NOT SO GREAT FOR NUTRITION

Environmentally, recycling is a great idea. However, in the world of nutrition, especially as it relates to weight loss and dieting, it means that if you are in the professional field for long enough, the same diet recommendations will just keep coming around. I have been in the nutrition field long enough, for example, to see the Atkins Diet (low-carbohydrate diet of 20 grams or less per day[1]) become popular twice (1972 and 2002). It didn't last very long the first time, but in 2002, Robert Atkins had a second chance and a whole new generation to promote his weight loss program to. With technology advances, there was also the ability to reach out around the world on the Internet and the ability to change food composition to achieve food products to meet the diet's guidelines. Add to this the climate culturally and even medically that stressed the increasing health issue of obesity in this country, and it was a perfect storm for his second chance.

Dr. Atkins was presented with a great marketing opportunity. Expenditures on weight loss in this country are in the billions of dollars annually. In fact, Marketdata Enterprises has projected that the total U.S. weight loss market is expected to grow 4.5 percent in 2013, to a value of $66.5 billion.[2] The recycling of the low-carbohydrate diet concept has been a serious issue in terms of working with students to become comfortable with carbohydrates. The National Academy of Sciences has set a minimum requirement for adults and children of 130 grams of carbohydrate per day for glucose utilization by the brain,[3] and the average person needs much more than that to meet energy needs, even more if he or she is active. Still the National Academy of Sciences minimum requirement is significantly higher than the maximum that is prescribed by Atkins's diet plan and many others that jumped on the same high-protein, low-carbohydrate bandwagon. Yet how many times I have I heard "I am a healthy eater, I try to limit my carbohydrates." It will take much longer to undo the damage done over the fear of carbohydrates than it took Dr. Atkins to have a highly profitable second wind.

NUMBERS MATTER

Numbers are concrete; they are easily used and accepted as a measure of success or failure, and college students are very aware of this since they often live and die by their test scores. Weight loss contests use numbers as a motivator, as a marker of success or failure. Weight loss programs have used points so you can easily calculate and control your food intake. The BMI is supposedly a number that tells you whether you are overweight or not. Food labeling puts several numbers on food packaging, now on the front of the packages to make it "even easier" to know what you are "supposed to eat," an external marker of whether you made the right choice or not, whether you are good or bad on any given day. I have countless times stood in one of the aisles at the grocery store and watched a shopper pull several items off the shelf to compare calories in each one so as to ensure he or she buys the one with the lowest calories. These are all numbers that externally tell you whether you are eating "right," have been "good" or "bad" in your eating, whether you should focus on weight loss or not, whether you are "healthy" (supposedly). Numbers are used to restrict one's intake, rarely used to increase it. In the work I do, numbers are one of the most powerful obstacles to overcome. The concept that one's self-worth and self-esteem are directly connected to what is found by the bathroom scale makes it difficult for individuals to stop weighing themselves, to give up the scale. Even if I challenge them with the actual science of what they need to eat—typically more than they are currently eating—I find it isn't the knowledge that they are afraid of or don't believe; it is the idea that it doesn't apply to them.

The students I work with see their world through high and low numbers. Higher numbers are sought for grade point averages, time working out, test scores, pounds lost, and money and protein intake. Lower numbers are valued in calories, carbohydrates, fat, clothing size, BMI, and the scale. With technology making it easy to keep all of these numbers on your phone, trying to get people to see themselves as more than a number is extremely difficult. Educating people that their calorie needs vary every day, that their health isn't dependent on their weight, that their internal cues can guide them better than any app can be like pushing a rock up a hill. Students aren't afraid of knowledge on its face; they are afraid that it doesn't apply to them. I always suggest an idea originally presented in the book I mentioned earlier by Geneen Roth:

A scale . . . is just a scale—a cold lifeless piece of metal—until we give it power . . . Throw your scale out. Or paste your ideal weight on it so that when you ask yourself if you are allowed to feel good about yourself that day it says "of course."[4]

You can have a good day every day!

THE POWERFUL MYTH OF THE FRESHMAN 15

You can't work at a university and not have heard of the "freshman 15" (defined by WebMD as "weight . . . that college freshmen tend to gain during their first year at college"[5]). Each fall, in anticipation of a new group of students coming to college, the campus paper will write an article or two about "how to avoid the freshman 15." In case you miss that, there will also be an interview or segment on television or another form of electronic media. It will even be discussed among incoming freshmen at summer orientation or with their peers as they are presented with a plethora of dining options in the cafeteria for breakfast, lunch, and dinner in the residence halls. Parents offer advice to their student heading off to school.

Some urban legends can be fun, make scary stories even scarier. Sometimes, though, you just wish they would go away, especially when they aren't true. Fear of this myth does a tremendous amount of damage behaviorally and psychologically as students make unhealthy decisions in an attempt to avoid gaining 15 pounds. What I have learned from 25 incoming freshman classes is that you have to know and respond to what people believe, not just know the research. For example, despite being in an academic institution, the research documenting that freshman students do not typically gain 15 pounds doesn't seem to matter.[6] This is because the fear of the "possible" freshman 15 (or any part of it) can displace logic and reason. I have counseled countless incoming freshman students who proactively lost weight over the summer prior to their freshman year in order to give themselves "room" to gain when they came to school. What they didn't realize is how this fear of what could happen can create for them a rigid approach to eating, the need for external control of diet and exercise, development of a disordered relationship with food, and possibly the beginning stages of the development and diagnosis of an eating disorder. The fear of weight gain, of becoming "fat" (by whatever the student's definition), can drive a student to disordered behaviors even more than the desire to be thin.[7]

Fear of weight gain can also lead to an increasingly negative body image if a student does gain weight. Nutrition and health literature frequently focus on weight loss or maintaining a specific weight. The truth is that not all weight gain in college is abnormal. For many, if not most individuals, some weight gain is normal. Adolescents are becoming adults; bones are becoming more dense. Factors that do change an individual's body including his or her weight are normal and appropriate. These are messages that students need to hear, and we attempt to get them out to students at Michigan State in as many ways as we can: freshman orientation, parent orientation, and activist groups such as Spartan Body Pride.

POWER OF WORDS AND HOW THEY ARE USED

There is an old saying most people know: "Sticks and stones may break your bones but words will never hurt you." Unfortunately, I have learned how untrue this statement can be. When I first started at Michigan State, I had a student tell me that as she was walking by a fraternity house, a male student stuck his head out the window and yelled, "You have a fat ass." She turned around and said, "Well, I could change that, but what are you going to do about your face?" Now, I don't think people should call each other derogatory names or yell derogatory comments to each other, but I often use that example to teach that we can internalize, personalize what others say about us, or we can believe in ourselves and not give others the power to make us feel badly. Unfortunately, words are powerful and there are certain words that for many create a negative sense of self: words about body size such as "fat," "overweight," "large," "obese," and words about food like "sugar," "carbohydrate," "fat," "dessert," "cravings." I have learned through the years that these words hold a rigid, narrow definition for many people; it is important to help people minimize the impact of these words on how they feel about themselves, how they let others make them feel about themselves, and how that impacts their relationship with food and eating, and even help them reclaim the words.

The word I have become quite sensitive to is the word "healthy" because so often it ends up being used in unhealthy ways. If you look up the definition of "health"—"the condition of being sound in body, mind, or spirit; a flourishing condition; a general condition of the body"—it doesn't say the definition of health is a certain BMI or a certain weight. It doesn't say that it is being thin, only eating fruits and vegetables, eating low carbohydrate or low calorie. What I have seen in the work I do is that "health" has replaced the term "dieting." When a student comes in for a nutrition session and says, "I am a very healthy eater," I am instantly worried: it usually means fruits/vegetables, low calorie, low fat or fat free, low carbohydrate, high protein, or some variation of those. It doesn't mean that they are meeting their nutritional needs; it doesn't mean they are indeed a "healthy" eater as I originally learned the definition of it; it means that they are dieting.

As described by Dr. Karin Katrina on the National Eating Disorder website, "Those who have an 'unhealthy obsession' with otherwise healthy eating may be suffering from 'orthorexia nervosa,' a term which literally means 'fixation on righteous eating.' "[8] Orthorexia starts out as an innocent attempt to eat more healthfully, but orthorexics become fixated on food quality and purity. They become consumed with what and how much to eat, and how to deal with "slip-ups." An iron-clad will is needed to maintain this rigid eating style, and every day is seen as a chance to eat right, be "good," rise above others in dietary prowess.

There is swift self-punishment if temptation wins (usually through stricter eating, fasts, and exercise). Self-esteem becomes wrapped up in the purity of orthorexics' diet and they sometimes feel superior to others, especially in regard to food intake. I have seen the start of this relationship with food and body time and time again. As professionals we have to be very careful how we approach nutrition, and how we teach and promote health, to ensure that we don't create more problems by reinforcing and celebrating, rewarding, unnecessary restriction and rigid relationships with food and body. In my work, I have replaced the term "healthy eating" with "positive eating," asking the students I see, "How can I help you create a positive relationship with food and body?"

PERMISSION TO EAT

When I received my master's degree I never dreamed that I would spend so much time telling people that it is okay to eat. For many people the idea of giving themselves permission to eat and to eat all or any foods is truly scary. The "theys," the powerfully negative words, the recycling of dieting recommendations, and the fear of fat have created a fear of allowing themselves to "just eat." Students will often come in and say, "Just tell me what I am supposed to eat!" They want to be told exactly what to eat in what amount to weigh what they want to weigh, to have muscle but no body fat, to never gain weight, to get closer to an arbitrary stereotype of beauty and health. They have little or no internal recognition and no trust in their body's cues for hunger, appetite, and satiety. I once gave a presentation to incoming resident assistants where I shared verbally and in written form Ellen Satter's definition of normal eating. Afterward, a male resident assistant came up to me and said, "This makes eating sound like it could be fun." Eating should be fun; it should be pleasurable. It isn't that nutrition isn't important—of course it is—it's that nutrition is more than a rigid way to eat. What is important is to eat a variety of food over time, listen to your body and your mind, give yourself permission to eat, and most importantly, remember that what you eat isn't a reflection of your self-worth.

I think everyone should read Ellyn Satter's definition of normal eating; it takes so much pressure off "the right way" to approach eating and your relationship with eating, and eliminates judgment and fear based on choices for eating.

What Is Normal Eating?
Normal eating is going to the table hungry and eating until you are satisfied. It is being able to choose food you like and eat it and truly get enough of it—not just stop eating because you think you should. Normal eating is being able to give some thought to your food selection so you get nutritious food, but not being so wary and restrictive that you miss out on enjoyable food. Normal eating is giving yourself permission to eat sometimes because you are happy, sad or bored, or just because it feels good. Normal eating is mostly three meals a day, or four or five, or it can be choosing to munch along the way. It is leaving some cookies on the plate because you know you can have some again tomorrow, or it is eating more now because they taste so wonderful. Normal eating is overeating at times, feeling stuffed and uncomfortable. And it can be undereating at times and wishing you had more. Normal eating is trusting your body to make up for your mistakes in eating. Normal eating takes up some of your time and attention, but keeps its place as only one important area of your life.

In short, normal eating is flexible. It varies in response to your hunger, your schedule, your proximity to food and your feelings.[9]

ART OF REFERRAL AND NETWORK

Not everyone thinks like you do; not everyone believes what you do. I have learned to be careful to whom I refer my students on and off campus. It is the reason I have worked to develop a network of professionals in the area as well as around the country who embrace the same professional philosophy: a Health at Every Size approach and encouraging intuitive eating and positive relationships with food and body. It is the reason that I developed the lending library for books and videos. There used to be a Barnes and Noble bookstore across the street from the health center, but I learned quickly that if I sent students over to look for a book on nutrition, they would go to the nutrition and health section and find only books on dieting. I found that I would have to send them to the self-help and addiction section to find books that would actually be helpful to them. In addition, I always call and check on appropriate referral resources (when students' needs continue at home during breaks). I am a dietitian, but I understand and know that many dietitians do not take a Health at Every Size approach and, as such, are not appropriate resources for my students. Many medical providers do not embrace Health at Every Size, and sending a student to a provider or providers who focus on weight can set back any progress that the student may have made. I have been and continue to be fortunate to have a network of Health at Every Size practitioners to work with at Michigan State University.

CHANGING PERSPECTIVE IS HARD

This is true in work with individual students as well as work with other professionals on campus and in the community at large. As I mentioned earlier, no matter how clearly students know that dieting doesn't work and hasn't worked for them, they are almost always more afraid of gaining weight than they are of the possibility of losing too much weight and being diagnosed with an eating disorder. I also recognize how hard it is for professionals to change their perspective on their approach to health, weight, or nutrition. When *Overcoming, Overeating* first came out, one of the authors spoke at a nutrition conference. I remember a dietitian standing up and asking, "If I don't give out a diet, what do I do?" I also had this reaction when I refused to step on the scale at a medical appointment and the medical assistant said, "But that's what I do." This is a time to learn new approaches, conversations, words, behaviors, and patterns that actually help individuals achieve health, physically, mentally, and emotionally.

It has been a challenge. Despite the wonderful advances in understanding the psychological aspects associated with nutrition and weight, there has also been an escalating focus on weight in a negative context, much of it on obesity prevention and cure. With a weight loss industry that makes several billion dollars per year, there is certainly significant financial incentive and force behind reinforcing that there is not health at every size, that thinner is better, and that all people can be thin if they just try. Add this financial and media force to a vulnerable college environment where peers are highly influential, being in relationships is very significant, and external validation is seen as critical to achieve success, and it has been a daunting challenge at times to continue to press forward.

On a positive note, research continues to make advances in substantiating these alternate approaches and ways of thinking around weight, health, body image, and nutrition. Just as my approaches to health have evolved over my time at Michigan State University, I believe that it is possible for all of us to make the change. If we are going to create a culture that promotes a more positive approach, we need to focus on what matters, question frequently, pledge to never stop learning, and challenge what we know is not correct. I look forward to the day that I no longer have to retrain peer educators or conduct continuing medical education lectures about how "diets don't work," and that the eating disorder team that I am a member of is disbanded because eating disorders no longer occur. Impossible, some may say, but I still believe it can happen.

NOTES

1. Beverly Bird, *Meal Plans That Consist of 20 Grams of Carbs per Day*, LiveStrong.com, August 16, 2013, accessed March 21, 2014, http://www.livestrong.com/article/220004-meal-plans-that-consist-of-20-grams-of-carbs-per-day/.

2. John LaRosa, "U.S. Weight Loss Market Forecast to Hit $66 Billion in 2013," Tampa, FL (PRWEB), December 31, 2012.

3. Institute of Medicine, *Dietary Reference Intakes for Energy, Carbohydrate, Fiber, Fat, Fatty Acids, Cholesterol, Protein, and Amino Acids (Macronutrients) (2005)* (Washington, DC: National Academies Press, 2005), 265.

4. Geneen Roth, *Breaking Free from Emotional Eating* 2004 (New York: Penguin, 2004), 115.

5. Denise Mann, *Avoiding the Freshman 15: An Interview with Connie Diekman, MEd, RD*, WebMD, accessed March 21, 2013, http://www.webmd.com/diet/features/expert-qa-avoiding-freshman-15-connie-diekman.

6. D. Hoffman et al., "Changes in Body Weight and Fat Mass of Men and Women in the First Year of College: A Study of the Freshman 15," *Journal of American College Health* 55 (2006): 41–46; N. Mihalopoulos, P. Auinger, and J. Klein, "The Freshman 15: Is It Real?," *Journal of American College Health* 56 (2008): 531–34; S. Gropper et al., "The Freshman 15—a Closer Look," *Journal of American College Health* 58 (2009): 223–31.

7. S. Delinsky and G. T. Wilson, "Weight Gain, Dietary Restraint, and Disordered Eating in the Freshman Year of College," *Eating Behaviors* 9 (2008): 82–90, doi: 10.1016/j.eatbeh.2007.06.001; V. Provencher et al., "Who Gains or Who Loses Weight? Psychosocial Factors among First-Year University Students," *Physiology and Behavior* 96 (2009): 135–41, doi: 10.1016/j.physbeh.2008.09.011; S. Dalley and A. Buunk, " 'Thinspiration' vs. 'Fear of Fat': Using Prototypes to Predict Frequent Weight-Loss Dieting in Females," *Appetite* 52 (2009): 217–21, doi: 10.1016/j.appet.2008.09.019.

8. "Orthorexia Nervosa," National Eating Disorder Association, accessed October 10, 2013, http://www.nationaleatingdisorders.org/orthorexia-nervosa.

9. Ellyn Satter, "What Is Normal Eating?," copyright © 2012 by Ellyn Satter. For more information, please visit http://www.EllynSatter.com.

17

The Size Friendly Policy: A New Approach to Health, Wellness, and Rights in the Workplace

Jay Solomon

The question "Do I work in a Size Friendly workplace?" [1] is one that does not arise often enough in business and professional environments. Despite a dearth of hard data to support that supposition, the dramatic pay divide between thin workers and their fat counterparts,[2] the remarkable number of workplace weight loss programs in both the private[3] and public[4] sectors, and the fact that only a handful of locations in the United States protects an individual's rights based on height and weight attest to this reality.[5] However, asserting that businesses, managers, and employees should be considering whether or not they operate or work in Size Friendly environments begins by understanding what such a phrase means.

Defining the term "Size Friendly" workplace will be done through the lens of More of Me to Love (MOMTL), an online community and store for plus-size people designed to help larger-bodied individuals find what they need to live healthier, happier, safer, and more comfortable lives in the bodies they have today. MOMTL promotes size acceptance and the Health at Every Size[6] (HAES) model of behavior-based, weight-neutral health. As the cocreator of MOMTL, I believe that these ideas—size acceptance and HAES—are complementary pillars of creating a Size Friendly workplace. By evaluating the degree to which MOMTL does or does not successfully create a Size Friendly environment, its viability as a corporate policy, and its effects on employees, I will endorse the promotion of Size Friendly workplace policies at other companies.

HAES tenets and definitions vary by practitioner, but for the purposes of this chapter I have chosen to adopt those outlined by the Association for Size Diversity and Health, an "international professional organization composed of individual members who are committed to the Health At Every

Size principles."[7] These principles are delineated as "accepting and respecting the diversity of body shapes and sizes," "recognizing that health and well-being are multi-dimensional," "promoting all aspects of health and well-being for people of all sizes," "promoting eating in a manner which balances individual nutritional needs, hunger, satiety, appetite, and pleasure," and "promoting individually appropriate, enjoyable, life-enhancing physical activity, rather than exercise that is focused on a goal of weight loss." I have leaned on the International Size Acceptance Association's definition of size acceptance, which it describes simply "as acceptance of self and others without regard to weight or body size."[8] While size acceptance is in many ways an issue of civil rights and the HAES approach concerns, quite obviously, health—and civil rights and health should not be conflated—there is nonetheless a distinct overlap in these ideas that strikes at the core of operating a Size Friendly workplace: ignoring weight and size as ways by which to differentiate—and most precisely discriminate against—job applicants and employees.

As an employer, I know that there are many acceptable reasons to differentiate one person from another, to hire one person instead of another, and to pay one person more than another: qualifications, education, experience, talent, motivation, trustworthiness, etc. However, size and weight should not be reasons to discriminate against a person, hire him instead of another person or pay her less than another person for the same work, unless there is an immediately practical reason that can be openly discussed by both parties. Obvious or arguable exceptions come to mind such as paying a larger NFL defensive lineman more than a smaller one or a small jockey more than a larger one, but those pay and hiring differences, to be sure, are based on the talent and results of either athlete and not an inherent preference for his size, even if his size is advantageous to his particular profession. There are also practical size constraints for other positions that affect hiring. For instance, if a person who is three feet tall applies for a job at McDonald's but cannot reach the buttons on the back of the deep fryer, should McDonald's restructure its restaurant to accommodate this potential hire? Could a person who is too wide to maneuver between the seats in an airplane's main aisle reasonably be expected to be a flight attendant serving drinks? The costs of restructuring a McDonald's or an airplane to accommodate employees of every shape, size, and ability would be prohibitive or even ruinous, and the issue at hand is not in these practical exceptions (however unfortunate we might find them) but in cases in which weight and size—the overlap of size acceptance and the HAES approach—are regarded prejudicially and discriminatorily. It is in this majority of cases that larger employees are hired less often, paid less money, and promoted less often than thinner employees[9] that Size Friendly policies are essential. Because size, weight, and height are not legally protected against discrimination in the same way that race, gender, religion, and other characteristics are, it is crucial to have an overtly stated size and weight non-discrimination policy—part of a Size Friendly approach—if a company wishes to treat all people fairly.

MOMTL is a unique case study in how to operate a Size Friendly workplace because its mission is "to understand, serve and satisfy the needs of bigger-bodied people, both physically and emotionally";[10] yet with size acceptance at the core of such a mission, it would be nearly impossible to fulfill the company's stated purpose if employees were not made to feel that their sizes and weights were accepted and respected no matter where they fell on the spectrum of thin to fat. Setting aside the fact that treating people in a size-neutral way is the right way to treat them, the company would be hypocritical if its size acceptance mission toward customers and members was not internalized as a Size Friendly workplace for employees. Even though most businesses' purposes do not exclusively concern larger people, creating Size Friendly workplaces is still important—if not more so, since discussion of these issues is not part of the business. When run optimally, a Size Friendly policy and workplace have positive effects on the mental, social, and physical well-being of employees, all of which translate into a better work environment, greater employee satisfaction, and higher employee retention. It has been shown elsewhere that each of these factors positively affects customer satisfaction and profits,[11] so demonstrating the validity of a Size Friendly workplace begins with connecting such a policy with employee satisfaction.[12]

I have interviewed MOMTL's six full-time employees, asking them 40 questions about size acceptance, the HAES concept, their perceptions and understanding of both, as well as how they believe those ideas factor into their employment at MOMTL, previous jobs, and potential future jobs. In addition, employees were asked 27 questions based on a numerical scale of one to five, with one being "strongly disagree" and five being "strongly agree" (three was "neither agree nor disagree"). Table 17.1 represents the responses to the numerically graded questions and has been incorporated here for reference.

While these interviews are not meant to be a formalized and exhaustive study designed to prove the perfection of Size Friendly workplaces, an evaluation of them is meant to demonstrate the value of operating a Size Friendly workplace and the positive effects doing so can have on employees' mental, emotional, and physical well-being as well as their job satisfaction and overall happiness and self-image. At the same time, I hope to demonstrate the viability of using MOMTL's policy of being a Size Friendly workplace as a model for other businesses wishing to employ a comparable approach. That said, after reading these interviews and evaluating MOMTL's employee remarks, it is clear that there is room for improvement in the way MOMTL manifests being a Size Friendly workplace in comparison to my perceptions of this ideal.[13] Analyzing those necessary improvements is crucial. Finally, for comparison,

TABLE 17.1   Numerical Survey Taken by Six More of Me to Love Employees in March 2013

How Much Do You Agree or Disagree?	Average Numerical Response
I am more likely to go on a diet since working at MOMTL.	1
I think dieting leads to a better appearance.	1.4
I think dieting leads to better health. ·	1.6
I think my employer cares about my body size/weight.	1.6
I care what other people think about my health.	1.8
I care about my significant other's weight.	2
I learn about nutrition at MOMTL.	2.4
My food choices are healthier since working at MOMTL and because of MOMTL.	2.6
I learn about the mental component of health at MOMTL.	2.8
I care what other people think about my weight.	3
I feel bad when I make unhealthy food choices.	3
I care about my family members' weight.	3.2
I care what other people think about my body.	3.2
I learn about health at MOMTL.	3.4
I learn about body movement at MOMTL.	3.4
I enjoy eating healthy foods.	3.8
MOMTL promotes customers' health?	3.8
MOMTL promotes employees' health?	3.8
I care about my weight.	4
The Health at Every Size concept promotes health.	4.2
MOMTL promotes community members' health.	4.4
Size acceptance promotes health.	4.5
I think my employer cares about my health.	4.6
I care about my health.	4.8
Size Acceptance promotes good body image.	4.8
I care about my significant other's health.	5
I care about my family members' health.	5
Average Age of Respondents	26.6

I have included the comments of a woman named Margaret Hollis,[14] who, when she filled out the survey, was not a full-time employee of MOMTL; however, Margaret has been a part of the MOMTL Community and Store as a blogger and customer for years, she is now a part-time MOMTL employee, she identifies as fat, and her extensive job history sheds light on what it is to be a fat woman in a workforce that lacks Size Friendly policies.

The opening short-answer questions of the survey asked about each person's understanding of what size acceptance and the HAES concept meant because, as all employees indicated, none of them had heard of either idea before working at MOMTL. Based on their responses, every employee understood the HAES model, which in their estimation included such observations as, "The HAES movement encourages a focus on actual healthy behaviors— eating well, enjoyment of movement/exercise—as a way to improve health,"[15] and "Weight does not determine how healthy you are." Moreover, when asked how they understood size acceptance, not only did employees grasp the concept, but also two-thirds of respondents extended the definition of size acceptance to include not discriminating against people based on their size (which many claimed later they no longer do now that they work at MOMTL). Rebecca said, "Size Acceptance is the idea that no matter what size an individual is, she should be accepted into society how she is. . . . Size Acceptance is also . . . not discriminating against someone because of how much she weighs and her size." To whatever degree each person's understanding of these ideas was nuanced, each response made it clear that the employee understood both size acceptance and the HAES idea and that answers to forthcoming questions would be well grounded. Since these notions are pillars of a Size Friendly workplace, the fact that all employees understood them, at least definitionally, bodes well. While it remains that for some employees these ideas lack a significant effect on their own lives—an area for improvement in the model and policy—it is nonetheless important that everyone working at MOMTL understands and has thought about these foundational notions.

In order to better understand how employees in a Size Friendly workplace think differently about themselves, their bodies, and their health in such an environment, it was important to establish their thoughts about previous workplaces that lacked such policies.[16] While the men had not felt discriminated against in previous jobs, both Jamie and Rebecca felt uncomfortable in the past because of their bodies. "I have certainly felt out of place in some work environments due to my size," Jamie commented, and "I have felt discriminated against in a workplace because of my body." Rebecca noted a brief time spent as a cocktail waitress where "how much money you made was not based off of experience and your customer service abilities; it was based on how you looked." As young women aged 24 and 22 respectively, both Jamie's and Rebecca's work histories are comparatively short, and that both felt this way makes it unsurprising that Margaret, a 55-year-old woman of size with a long work history, also felt discriminated against at previous jobs.

As a professor of nutrition, Margaret received nasty comments in her student evaluations about being fat and believes that "student comments made it evident that my weight was a major factor [in my severance]. I personally felt that my weight colored their opinion [about] my teaching" about nutrition. As if to reinforce their experiences, a thinner MOMTL employee, Ashley, noted that being small "has usually been helpful in my previous workplaces," and another smaller woman in her mid-twenties, Donna, wrote that she had "never felt discriminated against." Without harping on what constitutes discrimination, at the very least these comments illustrate people's discomfort that made their jobs unpleasant (indeed, Rebecca quit the cocktail waitress job almost immediately, and Margaret was fired, as her boss explained, due to her student evaluations, which she knew explicitly referenced her size).[17] It is challenging to recognize the tacitly acceptable behavior within environments that makes employees uncomfortable when a policy of Size Friendliness is not stated directly; but had it been clear to all employees and managers that no one should be made to feel uncomfortable because of her size—a teaching of any Size Friendly policy—then situations like those mentioned above could have been avoided or at least been cause for conversation.

Coworkers' behavior, the way one is treated by management, and what constitutes permissible workplace conversation also affect an employee's comfort within her environment. Jamie explained how her manager at a previous job dressed provocatively in "tight and revealing clothing" and flirted excessively with her younger male staff; Jamie observed this flirtatious behavior and overheard "the more salacious, obscene whispers" of her colleagues, which made "me feel uncomfortable about myself . . . since I did not dress as provocatively, and I felt sort of 'frumpy' in comparison." She recalled another "generally disliked supervisor [who was] called fat, a slob, etc. for his size. . . . People wouldn't hesitate to refer to his body size when they mocked or insulted him behind his back." Another supervisor was described by her coworkers as being "so cute in the face. She'd be really beautiful if she lost some weight." While this discrimination was not against Jamie directly, working in an environment like that—one that allowed these kinds of remarks about coworkers and supervisors—made her uncomfortable.

This kind of public conversation could be equated to discussing someone's race or religion negatively in the same context. Race, religion, and size have little or nothing to do with one's ability to perform most jobs satisfactorily, and discussing them in the workplace only serves to make other employees uncomfortable about themselves and the way that their own size (or religion or race) might affect their employment or their colleagues' perceptions of them. While the survey did not ask a numerical question about how much people cared what others thought of their body size and weight before working at MOMTL, employees' current average evaluation of the question "I care what other people think about my body size/weight" was a 1.6, leaning between "disagree" and "strongly disagree."[18] While they no longer work in an environment where this kind of talk occurs, as they all indicate,[19] MOMTL hopes that working in a Size Friendly workplace has made them care less about others' thoughts about their body size and weight and that this fortitude will remain with them at future jobs.

Like Jamie, both Donna and Rebecca relayed time spent at restaurant jobs that was made uncomfortable by other employees' body-related behavior. According to Donna, one waitress dressed "rather inappropriately, really short shorts and low cut tops," in order to "bring in more tips." While that is common, when compared to Rebecca's experience of being put "in the back of the restaurant in a different outfit while the smaller women (around a size three) were able to serve the front of the restaurant and the bar due to the fact that they had more 'desirable' and 'marketable' bodies (as my boss described it word-for-word)," it is hard not to see the latter approach as discrimination. Donna's coworker's individual decision to be flirtatious for better tips is different from Rebecca's manager's decision to punish her for not being "sufficiently sexy," and it is in these latter cases that protecting a worker's rights becomes paramount. In the absence of such legal protection, individual companies' Size Friendly policies become an employee's only recourse. It is unfortunate that our culture reinforces Rebecca's experiences as profitable to her company,[20] but we know why this happens, and many restaurants are built on such a model.[21] Because of this and since size and weight are not protected classifications under the law, in distinction to race, religion, gender, nationality, etc., employers and companies should adopt policies that protect workers from feeling like their bodies have anything to do with their employment.[22]

Making employees feel uncomfortable does not stop here but extends to the widespread conversation about diets and dieting. "Diet talk is pervasive," Margaret writes. "It's everywhere. It's almost impossible to be around other people without hearing diet talk." When serving as a running specialist at a sporting goods store, Rebecca was repeatedly talked to about losing weight, and "according to my superior, Running Specialists needed to 'look the part.' We were dressed in running attire, but I needed to be smaller. It made me feel very insignificant, and I promptly turned in my two-weeks notice." Both Jeff and Jamie overheard diet talk by colleagues at previous jobs, and while Jeff "believe[s] they should be allowed to live how they want as long as it is not negatively affecting others," Jamie's remarks indicate how these kinds of discussions in the workplace do negatively affect other people:

> I definitely heard a lot of body-disparagement at my old office. It was a totally regular thing for girls to go on diets, "detoxes," etc. It was also very common for girls to say something like, "Gosh I'm such a pig, but

I'm going to eat this whole meal," etc, as if trying to justify their eating habits to disapproving lookers-on. In fact, at one point, both of our supervisors were participating in Weight Watchers together, so there would be a ton of point values talk, how many calories they were saving up for alcoholic drinks later, etc. It was definitely disconcerting for me, because I was not on a diet and I constantly ate snacks/meals in this office in front of my colleagues. I wondered if they were judging me based on my food choices, or if they thought I should be going on a diet. I tried to shrug off any talk that happened in front of me or directly to me, especially if I was eating during the conversation. If someone said something to me, I would reply something like "I just love good food— I can't give it up" and try to change the subject.

It cannot be underestimated how detrimental this kind of perpetual conversation can be to employees, their morale, their body image, and their comfort at their jobs, which is why it is so important to adopt the kinds of policies that discourage such talk in the workplace. Jamie actually felt uncomfortable eating in her office, an act she felt the need to justify to colleagues and bosses because of their diet conversations. While Ashley felt uneasy for different reasons, diet talk in the workplace was still a problem for her: "My co-workers would discuss how much they wanted to lose weight and would call themselves fat and look for me to react to their comments, which always made me feel uncomfortable. All I could say was 'just eat right, cut out junk food, and exercise.' I felt bad giving this advice because eating right and being fit have always been very easy for me." These similar experiences demonstrate that whether a bigger or smaller person, diet talk is neither healthy nor appropriate in a work environment.

Company-sponsored or -promoted weight loss programs are an increasingly popular approach among employers, and Jon Robison, a PhD and advocate of the HAES approach, explains that "employee wellness programs got a huge shot in the arm from the Affordable Care Act which promotes the increased use of carrots and sticks to nudge/pressure/coerce employees into engaging in worksite wellness programs by tying participation to the cost of their health insurance premiums."[23] This coercion is also a potential source of workplace discomfort, particularly for large employees who would prefer to abstain from programs that are weight loss driven but feel social and monetary pressure to conform. Despite well-intentioned but poorly executed government incentives, weight loss programs at work would never happen under a Size Friendly policy, especially since such programs might be viewed as discriminatory if not participating or being fat leads to higher insurance premiums or other punitive measures.[24] Alternatively, at a Size Friendly workplace, programs promoting healthy eating and a variety of fitness opportunities would be appropriate. While only Margaret recalled working at jobs that promoted weight loss competitions (many employees had been working at MOMTL by the time the Affordable Care Act was passed), Jeff mentioned some relatives' and friends' companies that encouraged weight loss. "My understanding is that companies encourage weight loss in order to decrease their own insurance premiums, not out of concern for employees' health. Therefore they are not concerned with whether the employees are losing weight in a healthy manner," he wrote. Opposing workplace weight loss programs under a Size Friendly policy may be seen as disregarding employer-incentivized health initiatives, but this is not the case.

The difference in approach between weight loss initiatives and those health programs that would arise under a Size Friendly policy is their goal: weight versus health. While I do believe that numerous companies promote health programs designed to both lower insurance premiums and have healthier employees for many of the valid business and personal reasons related to employee health, programs whose central focus is weight loss are rarely executed in a way that is good for employees or even, long term, for businesses. Not only is most weight lost ultimately regained,[25] but the act of weight loss and regain repeatedly, known as yo-yo dieting, has been shown to be correlated strongly with health conditions like hypertension, high blood pressure,[26] and other heart complications.[27] Companies engaging in weight loss programs, like Jeff suggested, may not truly be interested in employee health as much as they are lower insurance premiums, and they may actually be compromising employees' health—even if unknowingly—and causing increased body dissatisfaction, a predicator of poor mental health.[28] This is bad for employees and ultimately bad for the bottom line.

On the contrary, an HAES approach to workplace health, part of a Size Friendly policy, would be weight neutral, taking the emphasis off of employees' physical appearance and size and eliminating related diet and body-disparaging talk in the workplace that is likely to make many employees uncomfortable. Rather, such a policy would focus on healthy behaviors; this would, arguably, make employees healthier for the sake of their own health, happiness, and personal satisfaction rather than merely weight loss, which is tied disconcertingly close to the corporate bottom line. Both health and the bottom line can be goals, but when the latter is pursued without careful regard for the former, the effects can be worse for both health and the bottom line than most employers and employees understand or expect. As the most recent Towers Watson Global Workforce Study demonstrates, employers who receive maximal engagement from their employees—translatable as those who are happiest and most fulfilled in their positions—are those that promote physical, emotional, and social well-being.[29] This relates closely to the multifaceted HAES approach and suggests that such an approach is good not only for employee health but for the bottom line as well.

Notably, every single MOMTL employee interviewed said that before working at MOMTL, she or he had never heard of the HAES approach or size acceptance, but on average employees gave a 4.2 to the statement, "The Health At Every Size concept promotes Health," signaling a level of agreement slightly greater than "agree," and interestingly a 4.5—halfway to "strongly agree"—to the statement, "Size Acceptance promotes health." Considering their healthy skepticism of workplace weight loss programs' effects on health, this evaluation of size acceptance and the HAES approach is a positive indicator that employees would feel more comfortable pursuing health programs under a Size Friendly policy.

Unlike previous work environments that made some MOMTL employees— particularly the women—feel bad about their bodies or uncomfortable with the prevailing office discourse, staff answered the question, "Does the messaging MOMTL promotes make you think more or less about your body? Positively or negatively?" in an encouraging way. Jamie wrote that it made her think about her body more and "in a more positive way," while Rebecca noted that she has "always been very comfortable in my body so the messages here have only reassured those sorts of feelings." Donna's response is particularly noteworthy because she has lived her entire life with a serious chronic illness. MOMTL's messaging "makes me think about and appreciate my body all the time. Learning and thinking about Health At Every Size makes me feel like my body isn't flawed or broken because of my genetics. I am reminded all the time that everyone's body is different." Dave said, "It's made me think more about my body and in a more positive light." While Jeff noted that the messaging hasn't made him think more or less about his body, he also pointed out that he is distanced from MOMTL community-based messaging since he works in accounting; that employees less connected to customers and community members do not feel that this body-positive messaging reaches them speaks to a gap in the Size Friendly policy as it is instituted at MOMTL. Margaret, who by comparison is focused largely on the MOMTL Community, wrote that the messaging "helps me worry less about my body, but to have more thoughts about what I need to do to optimize my health." Based on these remarks and scores, a Size Friendly workplace improves body-related thoughts, a predicator of mental and social health and a benefit of such a policy.

MOMTL employees also voiced respect for the HAES model. Dave commented, "I think it's a wonderful idea/mindset. Ours is a very body-conscious society." Jeff noted anecdotal contradictions in his own life that make it "easy to see that outward appearance does not speak to how healthy someone is." Echoing this notion, Rebecca said, "I believe that every size comes with its own complications due to being that size. This goes for being thin and for being a large person. I don't think one group of people is exempt from the difficulties that come with being a certain size." Donna shared that "I deeply appreciate any approach to health that focuses on body and mind. I have always been skeptical of diet programs, so it was nice to discover that there was a concept/approach to health that doesn't focus on [weight loss] programs. I think I've always believed in Health At Every Size. I just didn't have a name or approach to associate my beliefs with." The only person outspokenly skeptical of the Health at Every Size framework was Ashley, and interestingly, she is studying to be a personal trainer. While she thinks that "being a larger bodied person isn't healthy and comes with a slew of health risks," she submits that "Health At Every Size is a great starting point. Realizing you can do healthy things, adopt healthy habits no matter what size [you are] can always be . . . taken further, which can help achieve a higher health level. I believe Health At Every Size is a great building block." In order to support what MOMTL employees are saying and demonstrate to Ashley or other skeptical employees that the HAES approach is more than just a good start, MOMTL and any company that adopts a Size Friendly policy should more actively promote healthy behaviors in employees and offer research and reading materials that support the concepts.[30]

The positive effects of MOMTL's Size Friendly policy are evident in remarks like Dave's, who said that "MOMTL's messaging makes me think more about my health and in a positive manner." Ashley wrote, "I think about ways that I can eat better, more healthy," and Donna said, "MOMTL has just made me think about [health] in a more positive way." Margaret has been motivated to be healthier by MOMTL's messaging as well: it "makes me want to take positive action toward behaviors that will improve all aspects of my health." One-third of employees gave a neutral evaluation to how MOMTL's messaging made them consider their health, but they agreed that the messaging is clear, particularly as it relates to size acceptance, which Dave believes "is at the forefront of every decision that we make" as a company. Jeff noted "that we do not have any discrimination in hiring or treatment amongst co-workers at MOMTL." In addition to believing that MOMTL is very clear on these concepts, employees gave an average score of 4.8 to the statement "Size Acceptance promotes good body image." When taken in conjunction with statements about their previous jobs, their understanding of size acceptance, and the resultant positive thoughts about their health and bodies, one could surmise that employees' body image, and therefore mental health, has improved under a Size Friendly workplace policy. However, while Ashley thought that the message of size acceptance "is conveyed well on our website through the on-line community . . . it's not something we discuss often," which sheds light on an area for improvement.

Policies and antidiscrimination are important, but discussing these ideas as a team would reinforce their value. A more thorough examination of MOMTL's Size Friendly policy and discussion of its effects on employment at MOMTL—or any company—is an important element of a Size Friendly policy.

In addition to generally believing that MOMTL conveys size acceptance effectively, MOMTL employees have never overheard or, according to their statements, engaged in diet talk or body disparagement talk at MOMTL.[31] Considering the unfortunate ways that this kind of dialogue made some of them feel at previous jobs, this is precisely why a Size Friendly policy is in place. That said, this raises an interesting question about diet talk in the workplace, which Jeff noted at one point he considers to be different from body disparagement talk. What is the role of a Size Friendly employer when it comes to discussing dieting in the work place? On the one hand, if people choose to go on diets, that is their prerogative, especially if they choose to do so despite being offered material on alternative approaches to health by a Size Friendly employer. On the other hand, if it makes employees uncomfortable to listen to diet talk, should it be allowed in the workplace or discouraged in a similar fashion to the way many employers discourage discussions about politics and religion because they can be incendiary and not contribute to a healthful environment? What should a manager do if he or she overhears that kind of dialogue? While MOMTL employees have not heard or engaged in diet talk, so this issue has never arisen, it is my belief as an employer that a Size Friendly environment will regulate itself, especially if, as Ashley insinuated they should be, size acceptance and the HAES approach are discussed more formally. Even if employees are dieting, they understand that discussing their diets should wait until they are not at work, where such talk makes other people uncomfortable. Having evaluated employees' comments about the positive effects of a Size Friendly environment, we must also look at the other side of the issue: the policy's failings. This can be done primarily through answers provided by Jamie.

Jamie believes she has become less healthy in her tenure at MOMTL. She pointed out that she does not blame MOMTL for this, even saying, "I don't think any of this is necessarily anyone's fault," but it nonetheless feels like a failing that needs addressing in any Size Friendly approach. After all, employees should feel healthier after working in an HAES-oriented workplace. Jamie wrote, "I think more about my health, but in a more negative way. I do not take good care of my body or my health, and MOMTL's messaging kind of makes me feel guilty about it." This is particularly interesting when taken in conjunction with her individual numerically scored questions because she strongly agreed with the statements, "I learn about health at MOMTL," "I enjoy eating healthy foods," and "MOMTL promotes community members' health," and she agreed with the statements, "I learn about body movement at MOMTL" and "MOMTL promotes customers' health." However, she is the only person who questioned outright the notion that MOMTL conveys the HAES idea consistently, and she scored the statement "MOMTL promotes employees' health" with only a 3, signaling neither agreement nor disagreement. She said:

> I think in theory our office is a HAES-friendly office, but we don't always behave in the healthiest of ways. For example, we don't always have healthy food options for Friday lunch,[32] and it can sometimes be difficult for an employee to take the time to get a healthy lunch option if she didn't bring something from home, especially because a lot of us are very busy during the day and we just don't have a ton of time to leave the office and get food. We also generally have a very sedentary office—most of us just sit at our desks all day and don't get a chance to move around a lot.

She said the following despite feeling positively about the HAES approach:

> I think it has the potential to bring a lot of comfort to a person who may have struggled with her weight for years. It is liberating to think, "Wow, my weight is actually not as important as people have made me feel it is," and actually focus on things that do have a direct correlation with health, like eating better foods and exercising for pleasure, not feeling like you have to torture yourself in a gym to be "beautiful."

In these admittedly accurate portrayals of MOMTL, Jamie has honed in on an incredibly important issue: in some ways MOMTL is talking the talk but not walking the walk.

Employees feel better about their bodies overall and, as Jamie pointed out, "it's made very clear that our work environment is a place of respect and acceptance, and if someone were saying disparaging things, I think someone would step up and stop it," but that doesn't necessarily make employees feel that they are healthier. Some employees feel healthier, like Dave, who said, "I am more healthy since starting work at MOMTL," but he attributes this to feeling that his life is on the right track and "so my mental health is quite high." Mental health is an undeniably important component of health, but as Jamie said, "I have quite enjoyed learning about the HAES movement and Size Acceptance, but I have not put in the effort in my personal life to follow their tenants [sic]." I have not been "eating as well as I should, and not exercising at all." Donna noted that she has maintained her health level, which when living with a chronic illness is the goal—i.e., not to get worse—and she attributes this to "being able to work around my physical and mental health. It makes taking care of myself so incredibly easy and stress free." This care for mental health and putting employees first is part of MOMTL's approach to health, but it is not enough. Employees should feel and be physically healthier too.

Jamie's remarks about the snacks, lunches, and breaks provided at work are an honest evaluation of the gaps in MOMTL's approach. While it is easy to offer snacks that do not spoil, like granola bars, pretzels, and goldfish crackers, part of putting employee health first is offering healthy snacks like fresh fruit or ensuring that people feel they have the time to get a healthier lunch or snack. A busy day can impede people's motivation to seek out a healthier lunch, even when they know they are allowed to do so, and when this is coupled with a sedentary office environment, the effects on employees are not positive. Effectively enacting an HAES approach under the umbrella of a Size Friendly policy would include encouraging employees to get up from their desks a few times a day to walk around, possibly outside for some fresh air, to stretch, and to get their blood flowing (notably, a program put in place after the results of this survey were evaluated). These seem like small ideas, and none of them is forbidden at MOMTL (or, I dare assert, most places), but proclaiming that one is an HAES workplace and caring about employees' health means going further than not promoting weight loss programs and removing diet talk from the company environment. After all, a Size Friendly workplace bolstered by size acceptance and the HAES methodology cannot be defined only by what it is not but must be appreciated and promoted for what it is. That means providing an alternative model toward health: a behavior-based model. This could be done through programs or by simple demonstration and leadership when a manager or department supervisor suggests a group stretch or a 10-minute walking meeting. Doing so with regard for employees' personal choices and with respect for disabled employees or those with limited mobility is key, yet ideas for implementation are limitless and cannot be fully addressed in the scope of this chapter (though suggestions for getting started are offered below). Suffice it to say that formally promoting employee health under an HAES policy is both beneficial and manageable.

Jamie's perceptions about discrimination are also telling. Creating a Size Friendly workplace ensures that discrimination based on size and weight are not tolerated, and overwhelmingly MOMTL employees said that they had never felt discriminated against at MOMTL based on their body size or weight—not the way some had felt at previous jobs. Donna wrote, "I have never experienced or witnessed any discrimination because of size." Again, though, Jamie's feelings are different, and as a comparatively larger woman than most of her colleagues, those feelings are particularly important:

> I have not felt directly discriminated against but I have sometimes felt uncomfortable with my weight. ... For example, during Friday lunches I typically eat more slices of pizza than some other people, or I always order a large sub. So sometimes I feel awkward about that. ... Sometimes the office is set up in a way that is uncomfortable—for example, having to squeeze into a chair in the conference room when it is packed with boxes.

While I have never observed Jamie's eating habits as being different from anyone else's, and people's survey responses lead me to believe that they are neither judging Jamie nor interested in her Friday lunch decisions, her feelings cannot be discounted. A Size Friendly workplace is one that, over time, would lessen a person's anxiety about such issues because of the body-positive, size-accepting values it conveys. If more discussions about the policy and its underlying belief system were conducted, as Ashley mentioned, perhaps such concerns would be alleviated over time. Jamie's observations about the physical environment, on the other hand, are ones of which I am keenly aware and for which I am responsible.

One of the first steps toward creating a Size Friendly company is evaluating how the built environment accommodates all employees. This includes providing chairs that are high-weight capacity and in some cases without arms so that anyone can fit in them, ensuring that corridors and walkways are wide enough to allow any body size to pass unobstructed, and taking into account other considerations about the physical configuration of a space. Along these lines, Donna recalled the preparations before moving to new offices: "When designing our current office space, things like large bathrooms and wide doors/hallways were important." Indeed, the special, extra-wide front door postponed construction on the MOMTL office by many weeks. Companies that are concerned with costs (and what company is not?) will have a hard time justifying the added expense of high-weight capacity office chairs and more space than they thought they needed in order to ensure adequate maneuverability for all. Despite cost concerns, Size Friendly employers must consider these factors when designing their offices and planning future development and expansion.[33] These accommodations are also important for disabled and wheelchair-bound employees, whose physical needs may be different than thinner and more "able-bodied" personnel's. In addition to the importance of making people of size feel comfortable, inclusively designed offices enhance all employees' experiences and prevent the need to rearrange spaces on a case-by-case basis, which disrupts settled employees and draws attention to the person perceived as causing that disruption. This kind of attention to the built environment early in the process of office design also reduces discrimination toward future potential employees because hiring managers need not consider the added expenses of one new employee, only that the employee's job-related capabilities need to be evaluated.

Despite these spatial shortcomings, the merits of a Size Friendly approach should also be assessed by employee perceptions of its components' effects on employees' lives. In Jamie's case, this is positive. About the HAES approach, Jamie said, "I believe it's had a positive impact. I feel that I am generally more positive about my body, and any goals that I have for my body relate more to actual health indicators rather than just to weight alone," and Donna added that it has "certainly influenced how I live and approach certain things in my life." Dave wrote that size acceptance has reduced his own once prejudicial thinking and "helped me be more accepting of people due to their size," while Jamie shared that "I have much more respect for my body and others' bodies." Donna said, "I find myself being much more tolerant in terms of size/weight." Rebecca believes that she's always practiced both concepts, and that MOMTL's approach has merely lent words to her thoughts. Only Jeff said that neither idea had affected his life much; but overall, the response to these questions was extremely positive and can be viewed as a boon for a Size Friendly employment policy in the workplace—especially one that deals with plus-size customers and members. Nearly all employees noted an increase in understanding and acceptance of other people based on their size and ways in which their own prejudices had abated by working in an environment like MOMTL's. Reducing size-based discrimination is at the core of any Size Friendly approach and is a distinct win for such a policy.

When asked whether or not they had considered going on a diet since working at MOMTL, every employee emphatically stated, "No," though two people mentioned that they had never considered going on a diet before being employed at MOMTL. Both Jeff and Jamie took this opportunity to note that they had thought about and worked toward having a better diet, but each meant the word "diet" in the sense of eating habits, not weight loss; as in most companies, a Size Friendly one supports healthier eating habits, and it is positive that the MOMTL environment encouraged this line of thought.

The following question may arise as an employer reads this article: "What can I do to create a Size Friendly workplace?" While an official program has yet to be developed, there are nonetheless a number of ways that a company can work toward fostering a Size Friendly environment and incorporating HAES principles into its own approach and health programs. The first and most important step is crafting and publicly stating a policy. This can be as simple as including height, weight, and size in the list of factors that a company does not discriminate based on; depending on applicable state and federal laws, factors like gender, race, age, and perhaps sexual orientation might be included already on such a list, and adding height, weight, and size is a crucial first step to implementing a Size Friendly policy. If a company is interested in a more specific declaration of its intents to become Size Friendly, crafting this policy as a separate employee right is commendable. This might be something to the effect of: "Employees and potential hires will never be discriminated against or made to feel different based on their size, shape, or weight. Violation of this policy is subject to disciplinary action." This is similar in effect to a fraud policy, which is crafted and shared for two primary purposes: first, because an officially stated policy is fundamentally a deterrent against behavior deemed unacceptable (e.g., fraud or in this case discrimination), and second, because this creates accountability in management by ensuring that it should punish those who commit the stated offense. Ensuring that all employees are aware of such a policy is also essential.

Immediately thereafter, a thorough evaluation of current practices and programming is almost certainly in order, and removing or modifying any programs that either actively encourage weight loss or that punish employees for nonparticipation is essential. It should always be remembered that an employer can provide any options it wants for the health of its employees, but under a Size Friendly approach, it is not within a company's purview to dictate how highly employees prioritize their health or how employees choose to pursue health, including their free choice to utilize or not utilize the options provided by an employer. Employers that insist on a prioritization of health ignore the individual component of health and incorporate elements into the workplace that have nothing to do with one's ability to perform a job. Offering healthy options is wonderful—forcing participation is an infringement on one's rights. There are factors and conditions that cannot be considered by an employer—and may not be a company's right to know—that might lead an employee not to participate in health offerings. For instance, an employee might get sufficient exercise at home, diet talk surrounding health programming might be bothersome to someone, or physical activity done during work hours could lead to getting sweaty and being uncomfortable for the remainder of the day. Further, for an employer to imagine that it is the decision maker for what constitutes health and healthy behavior for a large group of people is arbitrary. Therefore programs that punish for nonparticipation are neither Size Friendly ones nor following an HAES model.

It is important to remember that an HAES approach is one that incorporates not only physical health but also emotional and mental health. As such, creating options that address each of these areas of health is valuable. Two examples from MOMTL are a focus on what MOMTL calls "Move 10" as well as the promotion of a simple site called calm.com. Move 10 emphasizes trying to get 10 minutes of consecutive movement at least three times a week. It has been shown that simply walking for 10 minutes just three times a week is one of the best actions someone can take for her or his health.[34] Therefore MOMTL employees know that they can use their time at work to get in this movement. This is valuable in a few ways. In one sense, employees are encouraged to get up from their desks in order to move around, since sitting for extended periods over the long term can have negative consequences on muscles and cause back problems. When MOMTL promotes Move 10, employees know that they will not be negatively evaluated for taking breaks, including and especially when those breaks involve leaving the building and taking a walk. Of course, Move 10 is not fruitful for everyone. Some employees have said that they walk or run every morning, and others who work in a warehouse environment prefer sitting breaks to moving ones. Under a Size Friendly workplace policy, adopting Move 10—or not—as employees see fit is absolutely fine. That said, a greater emphasis on walking meetings has resulted from a Move 10 attitude and people seem to enjoy the fresh air and the movement tremendously—not to mention that the movement seems to stimulate creativity. For the mental component and for those who prefer a different kind of break, we encourage the use of calm.com, a meditation website that offers simple, guided, 2-, 5-, or 10-minute meditations. Stress, while often unavoidable, is taxing not only on individuals but on work culture, and aiding people in managing their stress is one way that we contribute to their mental health.

There are numerous other ways to foster a Size Friendly workplace that would allow a company to start experimenting with this approach. The key is often about offering a variety of options rather than focusing on any one "solution" as the essence of bringing health to employees. In this way, the approach becomes more holistic. For instance, allowing employees to customize work spaces that are more suited to their needs, including standing desks, ergonomic chairs, or exercise balls as seats, having a break room designated as "quiet space," offering fresh fruit as snacks in addition to the more commonly available chips, candy, and soda, ensuring easy access to water, a sitting area outside for access to fresh air, access to subsidized massage, an area dedicated to movement and stretching (oftentimes a gym at work is an infeasible expense, but some area where people can feel comfortable getting their blood flowing a bit), bringing in a yoga instructor or fitness instructor to teach basic desk exercises, bringing in a chef to teach simple and healthful recipes, and numerous other options besides are all Size Friendly. Each of these is a suggestion. No one makes a person healthy, but part of an HAES approach is recognizing that health is not a destination; and for those who choose to, there are many ways to become healthier in body and mind. Considering the amount of time individuals spend at their job, incorporating a variety of health-promoting options, whether nutritional or physical, mental or emotional, gives employees an opportunity to learn that health does not need to be a constant and consuming pursuit but a positive, habit-forming, and enjoyable part of their lives. Much of health is simply access.

There is an enormous amount of pressure on companies and employees regarding their relationship and employee health. This pressure comes from the government, from insurance companies, and from employees themselves, and too much of this relationship hinges more on size and weight than health. While health and productivity are worthy goals from all sides, it is the way many understand and measure health that is flawed and requires reevaluation. It can be challenging to strike the right balance about health between a company and its employees, but I believe that the best way of doing so effectively is by starting with a Size Friendly policy that supports a weight-neutral approach to hiring, employment, messaging, and health. While MOMTL's execution on these ideas certainly has room for improvement, employees' own remarks make it clear that a Size Friendly approach creates a more desirable work environment for them and that as MOMTL builds upon it, its employees will be healthier and happier. With additional research and formalization, a model like this would serve to improve other companies' employee health and well-being while better protecting employees from discrimination and the discomfort of working in what may seem like a hostile environment. Even without an emphasis on health, a company's formal adoption of a Size Friendly policy sends a message to employees that they will not be discriminated against for their body size or weight and that they should feel comfortable bringing issues to their human resources department if this policy is violated. My hope and recommendation is that as more employers see the pitfalls of practices stigmatizing current and potential employees based on their weight and size as well as the benefits of size acceptance and an HAES approach, they will incorporate Size Friendly policies into their own companies.

NOTES

1. I have chosen to capitalize the term "Size Friendly" as a descriptor in order to distinguish it as a single term throughout this chapter and not to confuse it with other terms related to size, weight, and health.

2. Timothy Judge and Daniel Cable, "When It Comes to Pay, Do the Thin Win? The Effect of Weight on Pay for Men and Women," *Journal of Applied Psychology* 96, no. 1 (2010): 96–112.

3. Fall Ferguson, "Workplace Wellness and Weight," Health At Every Size® Blog, Association for Size Diversity and Health, April 23, 2013, http://healthateverysize blog.org/2013/04/23/.

4. This is, admittedly, firsthand anecdotal evidence. When I visited the U.S. House of Representatives and crossed through its large dining area I found internally organized Weight Watchers program posters.

5. These locations are Washington, DC; the state of Michigan; Madison, Wisconsin; San Francisco, California; and Santa Cruz, California. For more, see

Dylan Vade and Sondra Solovay, "No Apology: Shared Struggles in Fat and Transgender Law," in *The Fat Studies Reader*, ed. Esther Rothblum and Sondra Solovay (New York: New York University Press, 2009), 169.

6. Health at Every Size and HAES are registered trademarks of the Association for Size Diversity and Health and used with permission. For more, see ASDAH's trademark guidelines at https://www.sizediversityandhealth.org/content.asp?id=159.

7. Home Page, Association for Size Diversity and Health, May 20, 2013, https://www.sizediversityandhealth.org/index.asp.

8. Mission Page, International Size Acceptance Association, May 20, 2013, http://www.size-acceptance.org/mission.html.

9. Judge and Cable, "When It Comes to Pay," 14–16.

10. About Page, More of Me to Love, May 20, 2013, http://www.moreofmetolove.com/community/about/.

11. James K. Harter, Frank L. Schmidt, and Theodore L. Hayes, "Business-Unit-Level Relationship between Employee Satisfaction, Employee Engagement, and Business Outcomes: A Meta-Analysis," *Journal of Applied Psychology* 87, no. 2 (April 2002): 268–79.

12. It can be argued that a weight-neutral policy could result in fatter employees, which, based on insurance premiums that so heavily value body mass index (a defunct formula that evaluates the ratio of an individual's height and weight), would create a larger expense for companies. Without walking too far down the road of this argument and discussion—another paper (or book) in and of itself—I would argue that a successfully executed Size Friendly policy, regardless of a reconfigured weight distribution of employees, would ultimately result in a happier and healthier workforce that can be evaluated by standards other than body mass index. And regardless of the bottom line, a Size Friendly workplace, I hope to show, is ethically the right choice.

13. I admit to the many flaws in conducting research in this fashion and wish to share some of those flaws so that they can be part of the record of this study. In the first place, these surveys were not anonymous; I knew who wrote what because people identified demographic information. This allowed me to incorporate evaluations about how factors like gender affected people's perceptions of the questions when notable patterns emerged. In addition to my knowing who wrote what, employees knew that their employer would be reading their answers, which undoubtedly colored those answers. MOMTL personnel know how much I value the ideas being discussed in this chapter, and they might have answered certain questions to please me, despite both verbal and written entreaties that they answer honestly, even noting the fact that I did not want them to write what they might have thought I wanted to read and ensuring them that no one's job would be at all compromised by what they wrote. These pleas aside, I noted one set of questions to which an employee's answers were outright lies; whether this employee believed the truth was being told or whether the desire was to give the answer that person believed I wanted to hear is beyond me, but this illustrates a flaw in the study (though it is interesting in its own right). In addition, MOMTL is not a large company, so these interviews were with only a half dozen people, hardly a statistical sample. What is more, the average age of our employees skews low (26.6 years old), which means that employees do not have much job

history against which to evaluate their employment at MOMTL. Reporting is also anecdotal, after the fact, and in response to direct questions rather than ones whose purpose is masked and would leave the answering party off guard. Moreover, the questions are far from exhaustive. Finally, other than one nonemployee, there was no control group for comparison. All that said, these interviews still serve as a preliminary foray into this topic and demonstrate its viability as one worthy of further study.

14. Margaret Hollis is a name that has been used to protect the identity of this contributor.

15. Jamie and Rebecca respectively. All interviews were conducted in writing on March 19, 2013, at the MOMTL offices in Atlanta, Georgia. In the interest of both brevity and anonymity, all employees will be referred to by a single first name, gendered accordingly. Names will be included intertextually for readability, and I will not add a reference note or interview details from this point forward.

16. Notably, not having a Size Friendly policy in place does not inherently mean that a company is Size Unfriendly, but the value of a policy like this as a top-down one ensures a ubiquitous knowledge across an organization that not only stymies discrimination but actively changes the way employees feel about their workplace. It is in this distinction that the comparative observations of interviewed employees are relevant.

17. Her boss did not say that she was fired for being fat, but Margaret's students said that they did not believe a fat woman should be teaching them about nutrition and evaluated her in an extremely negative way. While it was the negative student evaluations that led to her termination, the repeated references to her size led Margaret to connect those issues, even if the connection was indirect.

18. Notably, the awarding of a "3 - neither agree nor disagree" to this question that causes it to skew above a "1" was by Donna, who, as will be discussed later, lives with a serious chronic illness. When she is unable to answer disagree or strongly disagree to a question like this, it's because she thinks about it differently than most people do. She cares what other people think about her body size and weight because doctors regularly encourage her to gain weight in order to live better with her illness, but the way her body processes food makes this incredibly challenging.

19. While this answer, like the answers to all questions, has a self-reporting bias, I can confirm that I have never heard this kind of talk happen publicly, though I cannot be sure if it has happened privately between two people.

20. Which is to say that these girls may sell more drinks, add something aesthetic to the environment that keeps customers there and coming back for more than the food, or simply flirt sufficiently with customers in ways that reinforce this as their role and that customers like. Other reasons surely exist, but one way or another employers must correlate waitresses of certain aesthetic sensibilities with more successful business or so many of them would not hire these waitresses in such high proportions.

21. Consider Hooters, which attempts to argue against discrimination lawsuits by classifying its waitresses as entertainers who happen to bring food rather than waitresses, who cannot be hired and fired based on their bodies and bustiness.

22. Though it would be nice, I appreciate that this is an impractical request of more superficial companies, like, for instance, Hooters. In the same fashion, it would be

impractical to ask Best Buy to adopt a policy about kids putting down gaming devices and media consumption tools to go play outside for 60 minutes a day. However, for companies who don't believe that their revenue is intimately related to the shapes and sizes of their employees' bodies, encouraging the adoption of a Size Friendly policy stands to have positive effects on the lives and comfort levels of their employees. This is not to suggest that all companies should not be encouraged to adopt such policies, but part of a practical effort in this regard would be to "bark up the right trees."

23. Jon Robison, "Wellness at the Workplace—the Safeway Debacle," Health At Every Size® Blog, May 21, 2013, http://healthateverysizeblog.org/2013/05/21/the-haes-files-wellness-at-the-workplace-the-safeway-debacle/.

24. While some argue that companies have a right to try to lower insurance premiums by lowering employees' body mass index, people can have many reasons for wanting to maintain a high body mass index, whether medical, sexual, pride-based, or other reasons, and to force such an attempted change—especially considering the odds of failure that many larger people know all too well—for whatever seemingly acceptable reasons, is wrong.

25. Linda Bacon, *Health at Every Size: The Surprising Truth about Your Weight*, 2nd ed. (Dallas, TX: BenBella Books, 2010), 170. See also Pat Lyons, "Prescription for Harm: Diet Industry Influence, Public Health Policy, and the 'Obesity Epidemic,'" in *The Fat Studies Reader*, ed. Esther Rothblum and Sondra Solovay (New York: New York University Press, 2009), 75–87.

26. Glenn A. Gaesser, *Big Fat Lies: The Truth about Your Weight and Your Health* (New York: Fawcett Columbine, 1996), 62–67.

27. Ibid., 74–78.

28. Janet D. Latner et al., "Quality of Life Impairment and the Attitudinal and Behavioral Features of Eating Disorders," *Journal of Nervous & Mental Disease* 201, no. 7 (July 2013): 592–97.

29. Towers Watson, *Engagement at Risk: Driving Strong Performance in a Volatile Global Environment*, 2012 Global Workforce Study (New York: Towers Watson, 2012).

30. The MOMTL Community offers a great number of reading materials on subjects like size acceptance, the HAES model, body image, body positivity, and more, and it is perhaps for this reason that MOMTL employees gave an average score of 4.4, halfway to "strongly agree," to the statement "MOMTL promotes community members' health." Bridging the divide between the perception of this 4.4 and the 3.8 average awarded to the statement "MOMTL promotes employees' health" is an important part of ensuring that a Size Friendly policy is conveyed internally as well as externally.

31. Notably, this is a question to which I know at least one employee did not tell the truth. This employee actually spoke with me on multiple occasions about dieting to lose weight. While I do not believe this person spoke with any other employees and our conversations always occurred when no one else was in the office, this highlights the self-reporting bias that is inherently problematic with such surveys. This also calls into question the validity of other employees' responses to this question, though I have never heard any diet talk or body disparagement beyond this set of interactions, so I am inclined to believe these responses.

32. MOMTL brings in lunch for employees every Friday as a way of team building and offering a workplace incentive.

33. Every person need not be provided with a high-weight capacity office chair who does not need one, but the environment should be such that those who need one can feel comfortable asking, or managers should feel comfortable broaching the subject without the question being perceived as an insult (i.e., "Would you like an office chair with no arms?" is not nastily calling someone fat but simply a question about trying to make someone's life more comfortable). Recently, I hired someone who I knew would need a higher-weight capacity and wider office chair, and I apologized that one was not available for immediate use but assured her it would be provided. We discussed the importance of openly sharing deficiencies in the built environment, so that she and future employees could be more comfortable. In some environments, such conversations would be seen as insulting, but in a Size Friendly environment they are as innocuous as getting a vent cover for someone who gets cold when the air conditioning is on, despite the fact that other people are hot and want the air conditioning blowing.

34. See the video *23 1/2 Hours* for more information: http://www.youtube.com/watch?v=aUaInS6HIGo.

About the Editor and Contributors

THE EDITOR

RAGEN CHASTAIN is a trained researcher, three-time national champion dancer, and marathoner who writes and speaks full-time about self-esteem, body image, and health. Author of the blog www.DancesWithFat.org and the book *Fat: The Owner's Manual*, Ragen's writing has also been published in forums including the *Calgary Herald*, Democratic Underground, and Jezebel.com. Her work has been translated into multiple languages and her blog has readers on all seven continents. She is the body image and women's health blogger for NBCs iVillage and a columnist for *Ms. Fit* magazine. A leading activist in the Health at Every Size and size acceptance movements, Ragen passionately speaks for people of size and against the ill-conceived war on obesity. Ragen has recently spoken at universities and corporations around the country and is a feature interviewee in the documentaries *America the Beautiful 2: The Thin Commandments*, released by Warner Brothers in 2011, *A Stage for Size*, released 2013, and Ragen's *MORE Cabaret*, 2014. Ragen led the organization that raised more than $20,000 in eight days and put up six billboards and 10 bus shelter ads in Atlanta to counter a fat-shaming billboard campaign, and the Skinny Minnie petition, which garnered more than 150,000 signatures and resulted in substantial changes to a promotion by Barney's and Disney.

THE CONTRIBUTORS

RONDA BOKRAM, MS, RDN received her BS in clinical dietetics from Michigan State University and her master's in nutrition from the University of Wisconsin at Madison. She has been fortunate to have worked in an amazingly supportive environment where she was forgiven for teaching dieting initially until discovering the truth about weight and health. Besides being a passionate advocate for health at every size, she can be found enjoying her family and friends, good food and good wine, traveling, and as many walks on the beach as possible.

HEATHER BROWN is the director of the Office of Grant Writing and Publications in the University of Missouri's Office of Research. She has a bachelor of arts from Lake Forest College, a master of theological studies from Harvard Divinity School, and a doctorate of education in adult and higher education as well as a graduate certificate in women's studies from Northern Illinois University. At Mizzou, in addition to her work in the Office of Grant Writing and Publications, she serves on the Chancellor's Standing Committee on the Status of Women, the Advisory Committee to the Office of Undergraduate Research, the Science Communication Network, Mizzou Advantage Advisory Board, and the Broader Impacts Network Advisory Board. Her research focuses on the relationships between weight and learning in girls and women, the ethical and practical implications of conducting research with stigmatized populations, and motivation and barriers to success in professional development and adult education opportunities for postdoctoral students and faculty.

JENNIFER E. COPELAND, PSYD is a licensed psychologist at Mercy Clinic Behavioral Health in Joplin, Missouri, where she provides services for eating, weight, and health-related issues. She earned her doctorate and master's degrees in clinical psychology from the School of Professional Psychology at Forest Institute. Dr. Copeland has conducted studies on weight stigma, perceptions of size among health care providers, and the effectiveness of Health at Every Size programs for positive lifestyle improvements, and has presented this research at national and international conferences. Dr. Copeland has been recognized for her work with the Research and Evaluation Fellowship from Forest Institute and the inaugural Health at Every Size Scholar Award from the National Association to Advance Fat Acceptance. Dr. Copeland continues to be active in the size acceptance community, where she serves on the leadership team of the Association for Size Diversity and Health and hopes to continue her journey of challenging personal and professional perceptions of appearance.

JEANETTE DEPATIE (aka The Fat Chick) is a size acceptance activist, plus-size, certified fitness instructor, professional speaker, and personal trainer who has helped thousands of people who haven't worked out in a while (or ever) learn to love their bodies and love exercise again. She is author of the international best-selling book and DVD *The Fat Chick Works Out!* as well as an innovative iOS APP called "Dance to It." She has also created the acclaimed "Every BODY Can Exercise" program (EveryBODYCanExercise.com), and cocreated the Fit Fatties Forum (www.fitfatties.com) and the Hot Flash Mob Movement (www.hotflashmob.com). Ms. DePatie has served as a spokeswoman for NAAFA and ASDAH, and commonly speaks on the topic of Health at Every Size at community and university venues including Dickinson College, Cal Baptist University, and Chapman University in Singapore. She was recently featured regarding her speaking role at USC's Body Love Week on the *Katie Couric Show*. She has been interviewed many times on television, radio, and in print by many important entities including NPR, *Dr. Drew On Call*, Fox News, Al

Jazeera America, CTV, CBS News, the BBC, ABC News, the *New York Times*, the *Wall Street Journal*, and the *Boston Globe*. A prolific writer and producer, DePatie also serves on the national board of the Producers Guild of America.DePatie blogs regularly at www.fatchicksings.com.

CHERYL L. FULLER, PHD is a psychotherapist in private practice in Maine. Her interests include fat acceptance, Jungian psychology, and dangerous women. She is particularly interested in the issues of women's bodies, especially the fat body, in psychotherapy.

MARSHA HUDNALL, MS, RD, CD is co-owner and president of Green Mountain at Fox Run, a pioneering women's nondiet health retreat in Vermont. Green Mountain was founded more than 40 years ago to help women stop dieting and learn how to truly take care of themselves. In addition to overseeing a professional program that helps women establish sustainable approaches to healthy living, Marsha has made it her mission at Green Mountain to help women learn to enjoy food and eating again while successfully managing their health. This is an area she is personally as well as professionally versed in: Marsha successfully overcame an eating disorder brought on by dieting. A thought leader when it comes to managing eating, emotions, and concerns about weight, and a voice of reason for the last three decades in helping people move away from diets, Marsha serves on the boards of directors for the Binge Eating Disorder Association and The Center for Mindful Eating. An accomplished writer and speaker, she has produced curricula, books, pamphlets, and articles in consumer magazines and professional journals about the impact of dieting on eating behaviors, including binge eating and emotional eating. Her most recent book is *Eating Happy: A Woman's Guide to Overcoming Emotional Overeating.*

PETER E. JABERG, PHD is an associate professor at the School of Professional Psychology at Forest Institute and a part-time practitioner in Springfield, Missouri. He values diverse professional activities including conducting psychotherapy, psychological and educational assessment, program evaluation, teaching, and clinical supervision. He lives in southwest Missouri with his wife and four children. As much as he loves psychology, science, and teaching . . . these things pale in comparison to the opportunities he gets to spend time with his family, his church, and playing in the local community band.

JENNIFER LEE has a PhD in creative writing and is a lecturer in writing, literary studies, and gender at Victoria University in Melbourne, Australia. She publishes fiction, memoir, narrative nonfiction, and academic papers, and is the coeditor of a forthcoming creative anthology, *Fat Mook.*

BRITTANY LOCKARD is currently a visiting assistant professor at Wichita State University. Her research interests include the body in contemporary art and the intersection between gender, food, and morality. She completed her doctorate in contemporary art history at the University of Kansas, her master's in art history at the University of Indiana, Bloomington, and her undergraduate degree at Vanderbilt University.

DR. AMEERAH MATTAR is a clinical psychologist currently based in Sydney, Australia, and her qualifications include a bachelor of social sciences (honors) in psychology and a doctorate in clinical psychology. She has clinical experience in assessing and treating clients with a range of mental health conditions, and has practiced in health, community, and private practice settings. She also has a keen interest in the fields of disordered eating and body image disturbances, and her work has been featured in a range of media such as research journals and online publications.

ANGELA MEADOWS A biomedical scientist by training, Angela has always been interested in human health and well-being. She has a bachelor of science in biological sciences from the University of Wollongong in Australia, and has worked as a medical writer and editor, and most recently as a systematic reviewer in the Department of Public Health, Epidemiology, and Biostatistics at the University of Birmingham. Despite her knowledge of biology and nutrition, Angela spent many years struggling with her weight, often wondering what was wrong with her. Always trying to learn more about health and fitness, she qualified as a personal trainer in 2006, and completed a master's degree in weight management in 2011. During the course of her graduate studies, Angela became aware for the first time of a growing body of scientific evidence challenging the relevance of weight for long-term health outcomes. She stopped dieting, quit peddling weight loss, and founded her company, Never Diet Again UK. She is a Health at Every Size and size acceptance activist in the UK and has never been happier. Angela speaks at national and international events on the science behind Health at Every Size and contributes to a number of magazines and blogs. She is currently studying for a PhD in psychology with a focus on size acceptance, weight stigma, and health. In 2013, she organized the 1st Annual International Weight Stigma Conference in the UK.

JON ROBISON, PHD holds a doctorate in health education/exercise physiology and a master of science in human nutrition from Michigan State University where he is adjunct assistant professor. A former coeditor of the journal *Health at Every Size*, he has been helping people with weight- and eating-related concerns for more than 20 years. From keynotes to intensive training workshops to corporate consulting, Dr. Robison is available to help both lay and professional groups understand and implement health-centered approaches for helping people with weight- and eating-related struggles. You can learn more about Dr. Robison's work by visiting his website at www.jonrobison.net, and he can be contacted via e-mail at robisonj@msu.edu.

ASHLEY RUIZ-MARGENOT, MA is a practicing mental health counselor and a proud graduate of the University of Central Florida's counselor education program. She is inspired to share her personal experiences with eating disorder recovery in the hope that it will educate and empower others. Ashley lives in central Florida with her husband.

DR. DEAH SCHWARTZ, EDD, MS, MA, CTRS, CCC is a retired professor from San Francisco State University with a private practice in Oakland, California. With more than 30 years of experience treating eating disorders and body image issues, Dr. Deah's most recent book is *Dr. Deah's Calmanac: Your Interactive Monthly Guide for Cultivating a Positive Body Image*. To find out more about Dr. Deah's work visit her website at www.drdeah.com.

JAY SOLOMON, through his business, personal endeavors, and academic work, strives to create environments that are safer, more comfortable, and equal-opportunity for all people. As the cocreator of More of Me to Love and The Cresca Group, he works toward these goals every day in homes, corporate environments, and the automotive industry. He has a master's in religious studies.

PAMELA VIREDAY is a teacher, childbirth educator, speaker, freelance writer, and well-rounded mama to four kids. She writes at www.wellroundedmama. blogspot.com and www.plus-size-pregnancy.org, and has been published in Midwifery Today, Our Bodies, Ourselves, and the "Science and Sensibility" blog. She graduated from college magna cum laude, has won several teaching awards, is a certified childbirth educator, won a Size-Wise Website Recognition Award, and was a finalist for the 2012 Best Pregnancy Blog award from about.com.

JAYNE WILLIAMS is a writer and nonprofit management consultant with experience in education, workforce development, criminal and juvenile justice reform, mental and behavioral health, and other social services. She has a master's degree in Slavic languages and literatures from the University of California, Berkeley, and a bachelor's from Harvard in Russian languages and literatures. She is the author of *Slow Fat Triathlete: Live Your Athletic Dreams in the Body You Have Now* and *Shape Up with the Slow Fat Triathlete*.

SABRINA WILSON is a biracial, fat, atheist, queer feminist who thrives in activism that fully embraces the wonderful intersectionalities of human existence. When she's not working, dancing in front of a mirror, or trying to perfect cold-brewed iced coffee, she enjoys spending her time with her loving partner, cuddly kitty, and amazing family.

Index